Create Your Own
Health Patterns

9th March 1989

To Da,

Happy reading!

Love Lorna.

Create Your Own Health Patterns

John L Fitzpatrick, CSSp

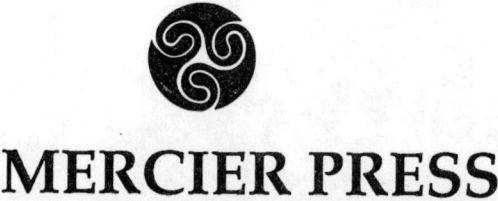

MERCIER PRESS

Mercier Press Limited
5 French Church Street, Cork
24 Lower Abbey Street, Dublin 1

© John L Fitzpatrick, CSSp

ISBN 185635 018 5

First published in 1980 in Brazil.

*To all who would like to enjoy better health
And are willing to work on it.*

No part of this publication may be reproduced, stored in a retrieval system, or transmitted, in any form or by any means, electronic, mechanical, photocopying, recording or otherwise, without the written permission of the publisher: Mercier Press, P.O. Box No. 5, 5 French Church Street, Cork.

Printed in Ireland by Litho Press, Midleton, Co. Cork

CONTENTS

Preface by Stanley Krippner 7

I: Development of My Interest in Healing 9
    The Awakening 9
    Brazilian Experience 12
    Healing a Disturbed Situation 15
    My Road to California 20
    Healing Experience 23
    A Healing Service 24
    Children are Natural Healers 27
    Carmel 27
    Regina 29
    Kathryn Kuhlman 31
    The Case of Jack Schwarz 34
    Belief and Experience 35

II: Why Healing Works – and Why it Doesn't 36
    Faith is Fundamental 39
    Jesus Demands Faith 40
    Hope and Expectation 42
    The Question of Lourdes 45
    Wrong Mental Attitudes 48
    Does God Send Sickness? 49
    The Importance of Desire 51
    Need to Find Specific Cause 53
    Salvation Means Wholeness 54
    Jesus Proclaims His Healing Mission 55
    Anybody Can Do It 55

III: Energy Transference and Healing 58
    Transmission Of Energy 62
    The Human Aura 63
    A Psychic Healing 65
    Laying on of Hands and the Aura 66
    Becoming a Clear Conduit 67
    Yoga and Energy 67

Celibacy	68
Fasting	69
Isolation and Meditation	70
IV: Non-Medical Healing and Medical Science	72
Inadaquacy of Medical Science	73
Some Unanswered Questions	75
The Future of Medicine	77
The Relation of Environment to Health	79
With Collaboration a New Hope is Born	82
V: Inner Healing	92
Healing of Memories	97
Forgiveness and Resentment	99
Healing of Relationships	101
Signs of Inner Healing	102
Conclusion	104
Acknowledgements	107
Notes	109
Bibliography	113

Preface

Paranormal is a term to describe instances of attempted physical or psychotherapeutic healing that cannot be described (or, if successful, explained) in purely medical, physiological or psychological terms. Successful 'paranormal healings' generally involve an unexplainable rapid rate of healing, or complete reversal of symptoms that is beyond medical expectations, or both. Assignment to this category is generally restricted to those cases for which a 'healing' was performed by another individual (priest, minister, rabbi, shaman, medicine man, psychic sensitive, etc.), a purported non-physical entity (deity, spirit, etc.), a group (prayer group, healing group, church group, tribal community, etc.), or by the sick person's presence at a place noted for miraculous cures (Lourdes, sacred tribal areas, 'places of power', etc.). In some cases the patient may be unaware that such a healing is taking place. A wide variety of techniques are associated wth 'paranormal healing', among them prayer, laying-on of hands, meditation, religious rituals, spirit incorporation, exorcism, and esoteric procedures for which there is no known medical validity e.g. colour therapy, special fasts and diets, music, dance).

The literature in 'paranormal healing' has been enriched by this volume by John L Fitzpatrick. He takes a holistic view that human beings are body, mind and spirit, and that healing must address itself to all three levels. It is not surprising that little attention has been given to the needs of the spirit in western medicine. But, asks Fitzpatrick, why is so little attention given to healing by the Christian churches? This is a critical question when one realises the importance of faith to healing. Not only does faith play a vital role in 'paranormal healing', but it is critical in western medicine as well, as is obvious when one studies the placebo effect. One's belief system is an important part of what type of healing one will find effective.

Create Your Own Health Patterns

Yet there is more to 'paranormal healing' than faith, belief and placebo effect. Strong evidence for the reality of 'paranormal healing' comes from a small body of laboratory research, some of which is summarised by Fitzpatrick. These data must be considered tentative until replicated more thoroughly. But in the meantime, they call for a major, serious research effort in this area.

While we await more definite laboratory investigation, one fact is clear. 'Paranormal healing', particularly in non-western countries and in developing areas of the world, provides a major holistic health care resource for society. These healers treat a wide variety of complaints with a combination of medicinal, psychological and spiritual curative procedures. The element of forgiveness is often crucial, and Fitzpatrick stresses how dropping one's resentments can be a powerful healing agent. 'Wounded memories' as well as bodily wounds can respond to the inner healing provided by many of these practitioners. And for those sick people in the west, 'paranormal healing' may provide a missing link in the treatment of stress-related diseases.

In other words, there are many frontiers of healing that both organised church and organised medicine have chosen to ignore. John Fitzpatrick's provocative book gives us insights with which we can redress this omission to the benefit of the world's patients and healers alike.

STANLEY KRIPPNER

Chapter 1

Development of my Interest in Healing

*The Spirit of the Lord has been given
to me, for he has anointed me. He
has sent me to bring the good news to
the poor, to proclaim liberty to
captives and to blind new sight,
to set the downtrodden free, to
proclaim the Lord's year of favour.*
LUKE 4: 18-19

The Awakening

As a child I experienced more than the normal quota of illness. In fact, I was regarded as the 'delicate' one of the family. I was constantly infected with all types of ailments.

Looking back I realise that my illness served a purpose because I was a home-loving bird and hated school. Later on in high school I suffered repeatedly from sore eyes and a sore throat. This often happened near examination time from which I was excused due to illness. At that time I was aware that it was serving a convenient purpose, but if anyone had suggested that I was possibly causing the infection myself I would never have accepted the idea.

My interest in healing began when I was eighteen, when a psychologist, Fr Bertie Farrell, visited our college. He had been a missionary in East Africa for many years, during which time he had carried out some experiments in dreams, clairvoyance and telepathy.

Later he lectured in the psychology department at Duquesne University, Pittsburg. During his time there he carried out some very interesting experiments on subliminal education among prisoners, which contributed significantly to their rehabilitation process. Though he was primarily interested in psychology, Father Farrell gained national renown in Ireland as a healer. His success in dealing with ailments, not only those ailments normally regarded as psychosomatic, such as asthma and allergies, but also such ailments as paralysis, arthritis and blindness, bordered on the miraculous.

In the course of his talk entitled 'Mind Over Matter' he explained the psychological principles governing mental and physical health. The occasion marked my life in some way, gave me a new understanding of health and sickness and generated in me an interest in this area which today has become a huge part of my life. It was one of the most fascinating and interesting lectures I have ever attended. The idea that one could cause one's own ailments or health pattern intrigued me. I became particularly interested in applying the ideas to my own case.

On the following day, Fr Farrell gave visual proof of the validity of some of his theories, with a practical demonstration on three asthmatic cases from my class. Two of the students had suffered from asthma since childhood and the third – a member of the college rugby team – invariably had a severe attack before each important game. After one hour with Fr Farrell the asthma disappeared and had not recurred up to the time we parted company as college students.

That brief exposure planted in me a seed of belief in healing that had been growing and although for the next nine years I had no further contact with healing situations, I became a strong believer in, and advocate of, some of the theories. I bought and avidly read any available material related to the subject. I began to think of the possibility of living a life free from all those ailments which I had come to regard as a 'normal' part of the human condition.

Towards the end of my seminary career, I had the opportunity to renew my acquaintance with Fr Farrell. I had been in close contact with him for about a year. During this time he shared many of his ideas and experiences with me. I had the opportunity to present some cases to him and to accompany his treatment of them.

Create Your Own Health Patterns

There is one case in particular I would like to relate here, as it is a very clear example of what one can do to one's body through inner conflict. This is the case of an eighteen year old girl called Bernice, who up to that time had enjoyed normal health. One day she lost her job. Lacking courage to tell her parents, she sailed to London where her brother lived.

Arriving in London, she failed to locate her brother and became very upset. Fortunately she was rescued by a kind lady who eventually got her on the plane back home to Ireland. A few days later Bernice developed some strange symptoms – a pain in her spinal cord, a violent headache and hard swelling on the right side of her neck. Due to carrying her head sideways she was developing curvature of the spine. When I met her, about six weeks later, the doctors were contemplating an orthopaedic operation to straighten the spine. At that time I understood enough to realise that this was a psychosomatic case, and dealing with the symptoms would hardly be an effective method of resolving her problem.

Fortunately I succeeded in setting up an interview for her with Fr Farrell. During the session, which lasted about an hour, the pain subsided, the hardness on her neck disappeared and she walked out of the office erect.

There is a sequel to this story which I must mention, as it has a bearing on something I want to illustrate later. A week after seeing Fr Farrell, Bernice was visiting with a lady friend, relating her experience. Her friend began to describe a similar experience that had happened to her daughter some years previously, adding, 'She also thought she was cured, but the ailment returned after some time and she has been in the mental hospital now for years'. Within a matter of hours Bernice had her symptoms back.

Fr Farrell agreed to see her again. He had one more long session with her and was disappointed at her slow reaction. However one week later she was completely well.

This example was, for me, a practical proof of the power

of applied psychology by one who understands the field. It also served to confirm my belief.

Brazilian Experience

In 1964 I moved to Brazil, where I had the opportunity of becoming acquainted with what was going on in the world of spiritism. This experience further stimulated my interest in healing. Though having a longstanding Christian tradition, the Brazilian people are steeped in the occult. Spiritism is very much a part of their thinking.

There are three major types of spiritism. In Salvador, the capitol of the state of Bahia, we find Candomblé, an old African cult brought to Brazil by the African slaves. There is Kardecismo, a Christian spiritism inherited directly from Alan Kardec of France. Finally there exists a Brazilian brand of spiritism called Umbanda, which is a blending of African cult, Roman Catholicism and Kardecismo. Candomblé and Umbanda are often wrongly referred to as 'macumba' a name used to denote black magic.

Candomblé is still associated with Bahia, but is slowly infiltrating the major cities in other Brazilian states. The spiritism of Kardec has developed rapidly in Brazil, and has a large following, particularly in the cities of Rio de Janeiro and Sao Paolo. The adherents tend to come from the upper and middle classes.

Umbanda seems to appeal to the middle and poorer classes of the Brazilian society. For some it is a religious cult, for others it provides a social outlet. For all, it provides a place and an opportunity to discharge emotional tensions.

Healing is an important part of all three types of spiritism, and each group has its own particular healing rituals. Estimates of the overall number of spiritists vary enormously, and it would be presumptuous of me to offer statistics. Many who believe in spiritism do not admit it, since spiritism has traditionally been condemned by the Roman Catholic Church since 1945.

Create Your Own Health Patterns

The spiritist world has produced some very exciting personalities, such as Francisco (Chico) Xavier and Jose Arigo.

Xavier, a famous medium, is revered as a saint among his followers. His speciality is psychography. (According to the followers of Kardec, psychography differs from automatic writing in that it is directed by a separate entity, whereas automatic writing comes directly from one's subconscious.) Although Xavier had never gone beyond grade school, he has written, through his spirit guides, over a hundred books, some of which are rich investigations into the nature of man, including a treatise on the corpuscular nature of the spirit of the psychosomatic body.[1]

Arigo achieved international fame as a psychic surgeon and some of his performances were truly extraordinary. He was a simple, uneducated man who claimed to have been in touch with the spirit of a (deceased) German physician named Dr Fritz, to whose guidance he owed his successes as a healer. He worked in a simple dwelling in the little town of Congonhas do Campo in the state of Minas Gerais. His operating table was a wooden bench and his scalpel an unsterilised butcher's knife. People went to him from all over Brazil and even from abroad. He performed all types of operations, sometimes using his knife, sometimes his hands, removing what appeared to be tumours, cysts and cataracts. He wrote out elaborate prescriptions as if he were a qualified physician, some for drugs no longer in popular use. His home had become a veritable place of pilgrimage before his sudden death in 1971.

Arigo achieved notable success, but like most healers he also had his failures. He became a very controversial figure, and many of his enemies still regard him as a fake, alleging that his psychic operations were done by trickery. If this be the case, they still must explain how so many people who visited him experienced a significant change in their health, while many others went home completely cured.

I lived in Brazil while he was still alive and I had ample opportunity to see him, but never did because I was a more biased Catholic at that time than I am now and Arigo was a Catholic turned spiritist.

From what I have seen of spiritist healing in Brazil I make the following observations (which, in fact, are valid for every healing group I have known):

> 1. Some people are healed of various types of illness, including grave ones.
> 2. Some do not experience any healing at all while others become even worse.
> 3. Some appear to be cured for a time but fail to keep their healing.

I would like to add that because of the strong emphasis on the intervention of spirits, many people are left anxious and confused, and end up graduating from the spiritist centre to the psychiatric ward of the hospital.

One may ask at this point why spiritism has such an appeal in Brazil. In general it responds to a need in the Brazilian people to which none of the Christian religions address themselves. Many turn to the spiritist centre at a time of financial difficulty, or when bad luck or illness invade their homes. I should also mention that the scarcity of doctors, coupled with medical fees and the exorbitant prices of medicine, are concerns which often leave the ordinary people no alternative except to have recourse to the clinic – in the interest of survival.

The Christian churches – to which almost all the spiritists are affiliated – have not been giving them any real effective help in this area, except for prayer and resignation. These, however, do not seem to solve the problems.

Finally I quote Frei Bonaventure Kloppenburg, a Franciscan priest in Petropolis who spent ten years of his life waging an unrelentless war against spiritism. After the Second Vatican Council he underwent a change of mind and a change of heart in relation to spiritism, and writing on Umbanda stated, 'We must respect, raise up and consummate in Christ everything we discover as being truly good, beautiful, just, holy and lovable in Umbanda. As the church has changed its attitude and mentality, so have I.'[2]

Healing a Disturbed Situation

Before leaving the Brazilian scene I want to share an unusual healing phenomenon. It was not physical illness, nor strictly a mental illness, but rather a disease in a home. It was what we would call in Ireland a haunted house. Some people would call it poltergeist. The exorcist would probably describe it in terms of a satanic presence.

Some years ago I had been given a theory which attempted to explain such phenomena as ghosts, poltergeists and the presence of evil. In Ireland the presence of ghosts and haunted houses has been traditionally accepted as a reality, and various theories have been put forward to explain such phenomena.

(By haunted house I mean a strange mysterious presence in the home, such as the sound of footsteps in the middle of the night, the playing of music, the sound of voices, and the shifting of furniture). The popular theory about ghosts or poltergeists attributes such happenings to the return of a soul to fulfil some duty it has failed to fulfil during life, or seeking help in some mysterious way from its loved ones. The 'new' theory, however, would understand ghosts in terms of our own creation, based on the emanation of ectoplasm from the human body and the projection of an image on it.

So ghosts are a product of the imagination, not a fiction of the imagination. They form a separate reality from the person causing them. A poltergeist in a home, for example, is not caused by strange occult forces but usually by one of the family living in the home, and it has been found that the person responsible is usually (but not always) a boy or girl at the age of puberty. At that age the imagination is at the highest point of development. It is very fertile and uncontrolled, extremely vivid and creative, and capable of producing unusual phenomena.

The poltergeist then can be understood in terms of the presence of an energy body created by a person. It appears to be under the control of the subconscious mind of the person causing it and can be made to interfere in all sorts of ways with people and situations. It is usually a symptom of a mild form of mental disturbance such as jealousy, hate, resentment or dissatisfaction with a person or situation.

In the particular case in question, I decided to work along the lines suggested by this theory. I take up the story as related by Guy Lyon Playfair in his book *The Flying Cow:*

> The Suzano case began with a bang. It was just after midday on May 22, 1970. Nobody was in the house at the time. Fifteen year old Irene was washing clothes in a neighbour's house when the loud explosion was heard coming from her home. Smoke began to peep through the tiles of the roof and neighbours rushed in to find that fire had broken out inside a wardrobe, burning holes in several items of clothing.
>
> The fire was easily put out, but at five o'clock the same afternoon bedclothes in the same room caught fire on each of two beds. Again, there was nobody around at the time, Irene being twenty yards away from outside the house.
>
> Less than an hour later, clothing that had been rescued from the last fire and dumped in the outside bathroom caught fire again, although it was still soaking wet.
>
> Later that night, the owner of the house was roused by screams and yells from the room where his four children were sleeping. A fireball, they told him, had come down and set fire to their mattress. Unable to put the fire out, they dragged the mattress into the yard where it was completely destroyed.
>
> Ten minutes later the sofa in the living-room caught fire. Water was thrown on it and the fire extinguished, but after it also had been dragged out into the yard it caught fire again, although saturated with water, this time burning itself completely out.
>
> At this point a police patrol happened to pass by, stopping their car to see what all the fuss was about at that time of night, for a small multitude of neighbours had begun to gather. The policemen offered to help while one of them put through a call to headquarters to report the incident.
>
> At the police station, the *delegado* on duty felt uncom-

fortable. Only a few days earlier he had received an official complaint from the owner of the house that stones had been thrown through his window and even through his roof, breaking several tiles. The officer had thought little of the incidents at the time, but now he decided to have a look for himself.

While waiting for their chief to arrive, one of the policemen picked up a calendar from the floor and hung it on a nail on the bedroom wall. After a few minutes it blackened and burst into flames. It was, he later testified, a bluish flame like that of a gas burner, and when he put his finger in it, he burned it as he would have done in a normal flame.

At that moment the chief arrived, and the policeman took a sheet of newspaper and hung it from a nail on the living room wall. This also caught fire, leaving a burn mark on the wall behind it, although it was damp when picked up from the floor.

The following day, another minor fire broke out in a kitchen cabinet, and five days later there were two more cases of parapyrogenia, one in the main bedroom (in the baby's cradle, which had already been attacked) and the other in the children's room, where a bed lent by neighbours to replace the one that had been destroyed earlier also caught fire. On both these occasions nobody was in the house at the time. The children had been moved to a house nearby for their safety. This made a total of ten cases of paranormal spontaneous combustion, at least one of which had been personally witnessed by a *delegado*, or police commissioner.

All phenomena ceased when Irene was sent away to stay with an aunt for a few days, at the suggestion of a local priest, whom the girl's mother had asked to come and exorcise the house. The priest refused to do this, so yet again the spiritists were called in as a last resort.[3]

I happened to be the priest in question. A few days before the initial attack of fire the father of the family had come to me complaining about stones falling on the roof of the house, and asked me if I would go and bless it. I was not particularly interested in blessing it because according to my understanding of the nature of the problem I did not believe a blessing was necessary.

According to the story the father told me, no one was throwing the stones, they appeared to come out of nowhere.

Create Your Own Health Patterns

It was happening at different times of the day or night and with greater or lesser intensity. Sometimes it appeared to be a shower of stones. The stones were of different quality from those in the area.

Some days later a young lady came rushing up to my door in a state of mild panic and urgently pleaded with me to go and bless her neighbour's house which was catching fire. When I asked her if someone was setting it on fire she assured me this was not the case, but that it seemed to be catching fire of itself. When she described the location of the house it occurred to me that this might be the same place where the stone phenomenon happened. It was.

By this time the stone throwing had subsided and the house, a small brick building with a red tiled roof, was now being attacked by fire. In front of the house was a small yard, littered with partially burned objects, mostly items of furniture and clothing. When I arrived, a large group of neighbours were present to witness the scene and the atmosphere was one of wild commotion.

Two handsome young men were just leaving the scene on their motor-cycles. I was informed that they were two Protestant pastors who had come the previous afternoon and had offered their services. According to their thinking the disturbance was due to the fact that the family was involved in idolatry, the adoration of images, and so they induced the family to get rid of all their statues, breaking them into small pieces. Then having prayed with the family, the pastors departed. But the disturbance continued.

Some of the local spiritist leaders, including a famous macumbeiro, the local voodoo man, were also called upon to perform their rituals but none succeeded in breaking the spell.

According to the story related to me the stones falling on the tiles had been going on for two years. Then at a certain stage the panes of the windows became the object of attack. Subsequently the strange presence actually invaded the house, breaking the glass in the china cabinet and partially

Create Your Own Health Patterns

burning the woodwork. The presence of the fire was the final stage as the disturbing forces launched their attack with greater intensity.

My initial step was to invite the family to my home. All accepted – father, mother, and five children. The oldest child was Irene, a highly strung and intelligent girl of fourteen; the next was a boy of twelve. Falling back on my theory I suspected the girl of fourteen was the one responsible for the phenomenon.

I was very interested in finding out how they related to each other. I learned that some years previously the father had been living with a neighbouring woman. At the time he left her (which was two years previously) and returned to his own family, the stones began falling on the roof. The family believed that the neighbour, in her jealousy and rage, was doing *macumba* on them (macumba is a ritual performed to transmit evil to another person).

Upon further investigation it became apparent that Irene had a very deep resentment against her father. First of all she had never accepted him since he returned to his wife two years before. The father insisted on her staying home every night, and never allowed her out with her friends. She had wanted to take on a job in a local factory but he forbade this. On two occasions she had run away from home, but was picked up and brought back by the police.

Two other interesting factors came to light. One was that when the wardrobe caught fire, the mother's clothes, which were on one side of a partition, got burnt, but Irene's clothes, which were in the same wardrobe, but on the other side of the partition, did not. The second one was when I asked the mother, 'How does Irene react during the actual fire phenomenon?' and she replied, 'She seems to enjoy it thoroughly'.

When I suggested to them that Irene was possibly connected to this whole phenomena and perhaps causing it, they were really shocked and wanted to know if she was possessed by some evil spirit. Telling them that this was a parapsychological phenomenon would not have meant much to them.

They did agree, though, to send Irene away to her aunt's house for two weeks, just to see how things would be in her absence. Two weeks later I called upon the family and the first person I met was Irene. She had returned the previous evening. When the mother appeared on the scene I put the inevitable question, 'How have things been?'

Her answer was, 'Well, to tell you the truth, Padre, we had total peace in the house for the past two weeks. Irene returned yesterday and the house caught fire again last night'.

At that point I took Irene for one interview, in the course of which I tried to get her to consciously accept her father, forgive him for what he had done, and let go of that resentment. Incredible though it may seem, that was the end of the fire, and as far as I could ascertain, there was no further disturbance.

This for me is an example of healing, of re-establishing harmony in a disturbed person and situation. Perhaps if the 'exorcist' had been there before me he would have achieved the same result, but by taking a different road.

My Road to California

In June 1973 I went to study psychology in San Francisco, California. As part of my course I opted to write a thesis on healing, and this automatically involved me in research on this topic. Within a short time I had become aware of the astounding development of interest in healing in the United States and especially in the San Francisco Bay area. Not only did I have access to ample reading on the subject but I also had the opportunity to get into close contact with some of those active in the healing field. I looked at and experienced a variety of healing approaches, such as spiritual healing, psychic healing, faith healing, herbal treatment, megavitamin therapy, body work and meditation.

Create Your Own Health Patterns

My first contact in the field was at a seminar on Pentecostalism in Oakland. Although I did not go specifically to study Pentecostal healing, it turned out to be the one area in which I became interested. The occasion was a talk entitled 'Healing Through the Spirit' given by Rita Bennett, a minister from Los Angeles. Rita has had quite a lot of success in healing and in the course of her talk she described some of her cases and how she went about healing them. One thing she strongly emphasised as an important condition for healing is faith on the part of the person ill. 'However,' she said, 'this faith is a commodity that is usually not present, due to the belief pattern in our present-day culture. It has to be built.' Rita went on to explain that she normally has a lot of 'ground work' to do before the sick person is ready for a healing. She believes that once faith is present, the healing takes place when the prayer for healing is made.

Shortly after this experience, I attended the Silva Mind Control course. This again added a little more impetus to my interest in healing and my belief reached a higher plateau. This programme, developed by Jose Silva from Laredo. Texas, is basically a course on techniques and exercises for developing greater access to the limitless powers of the mind, and utilising those powers to greater avail, for our own betterment and the betterment of humanity. Belief and correct positive thinking are two basic conditions for success. Silva is a strong believer in healing, but he believes more in living healthily – in living free from sickness. During the course, specific techniques were given for getting rid of headaches and migraine, low and high blood pressure, controlling pain and bleeding. Students had an opportunity to try to put some of these techniques into practice and see how they function.

At one period during my stay in San Francisco, I suffered from a very severe headache. I had been taking various kinds of tablets but relief was always short-lived. Finally it dawned on me that Silva Mind Control had given me a technique for headache control which I had never used for my own relief. So I tried, and within minutes my headache was gone. It has worked every time since, and I have never again had to resort to any kind of tablets to relieve headache.

Later I attended a very interesting workshop given by Helen Hadsell, whose thinking is influenced by the concepts of Wilhelm Reich. She spoke of the control of energy through mental power and its use for various purposes including healing. In her book called *The Name It and Claim It Game*[4] she tells of the amazing events in her life that bear out her conviction that anyone can achieve extraordinary results through the correct use of the mind.

Helen holds the unique record of having submitted a winning entry in every contest she ever entered. Her prizes since the beginning of her contest career have included sports equipment, electric appliances, a Hammond organ and trips to New York, Washington and Europe. In 1966 she won a $50,000 home. By way of explanation of her good fortune she stated, 'I don't believe in luck and I don't believe in accidents. I project my goal in my mind's eye and then I give it nothing but positive energy'. The basic premise on which she builds her whole philosophy is one borrowed from Norman Vincent Peale, author of *The Power of Positive Thinking*, and it reads, 'Whatever the mind can conceive and believe, it can achieve'.[5]

Helen is a graduate of Silva Mind Control. Although she had been into the winning game long before she took Silva's course, she states that she really improved her ability after taking the course. She came from a German Catholic background where illness was often seen as coming from the hand of God and must be borne with patience and resignation. On the other hand, her mother had such a terrific fear of illness and so scared her children about the possibility of catching illness that they ended up catching all the ailments imaginable. Helen learned from this, and through many years of working at it, she reversed her thinking patterns and became a very healthy person.

A few years ago she and her husband were involved in

an automobile accident. She was thrown against the dashboard and sustained severe injuries including a broken nose, fractured ribs, a broken ankle and bruised spleen. Due to the great amount of blood she was swallowing she was unable to breathe. At that moment she had two choices – to push the panic button and bleed to death or stop the bleeding. Using one of the techniques she learned in Silva Mind Control, she stopped the bleeding. By imagining all those throbbing pains as energy vibrations bringing healing, she succeeded in controlling the pain and made it to the hospital two hours later.

She had to have her face rebuilt through plastic surgery and was told by her doctors that the restoration process would take six weeks. Two weeks later she requested the doctors to remove the dressing. They refused. Even her husband could not prevail upon them to do it, and it was only when threatened by her lawyer that they acceded to her request. To their amazement her face was completely healed, and to use her own words her nose 'is running perfectly til this day.'

My contact with Helen reinforced my belief in the possibility of healing, a belief that is not normally held by people in our technologically orientated society.

Subsequently I assisted a number of workshops on healing techniques directed by Betty Bethards. In recent years Betty had become famous in California as a healer. She classifies herself as a psychic healer, emphasising the importance of daily meditation as an aid to healing, and uses the laying on of hands. She understands the healing process as a transference of energy from the healer to the healee. The energy comes from God, and the healer is merely a channel or conduit.

Healing Experience

The sacrament of Anointing has been used in the Roman Catholic Church for centuries to prepare those who were seriously ill to confront death, thus enabling them to make a satisfactory transition. This, for me, was an ill use or rather an abuse of the sacrament, defeating the whole purpose for which the sacrament was instituted. This abuse reached its highest point in Brazil, where the practice prevails of allowing the sick to enter a coma before the priest is called. According to their rationale the presence of the priest with his anointing kit indicates certain death and so he is called upon only when the last ray of hope for recovery has died. Also, once the sick person is in an unconscious state, he is spared the 'frightening' experience of the presence of the priest.

Needless to say this whole approach helped to undermine my belief in the anointing of the sick. The final blow came – which for me became a moment of decision – when on one occasion I was called at about two o'clock in the morning to anoint on of the members of the town council. There was a state car waiting at my doorstep. On my way I inquired of the chauffeur if this man had taken ill suddenly. He informed me that the man had been ill for the past week, and added, 'You know how it is, Father, these people did not want to upset him by calling the padre to perform the last rites. When he became unconscious about an hour ago they thought it would be safe to call you.'

That was something I needed to hear. Though I had been conscious of such a mentality for a long time, hearing it expressed in so many words jolted me into taking a stand. From then on, I began working towards giving the sacrament the meaning it was originally intended to have and to use it in the context of healing the sick.

A Healing Service

My first public healing service was at St John's Church in San Lorenzo, California. It was basically the application of the sacrament of Anointing the Sick, in the form of a communal service incorporated into the Sunday liturgy. The prim-

Create Your Own Health Patterns

ary purpose of the service was to restore the sick to better health. I also saw it as a faithbuilding experience through which the people's faith in healing might be rekindled or strengthened. It also served as an opportunity for people to readjust their thinking in relation to the use of the sacrament of Anointing and perhaps see it in a more positive light.

On the Sunday prior to the healing service I spoke at all seven Masses and reached perhaps four thousand people. It was an attempt to renew the people's belief in the possibility of healing, emphasising the fact that man is meant to be healthy.

The service was attended by about 800 people of all ages and suffering from various illnesses. I explained that sickness included not only the usual physical and mental ailments with which we are all very familiar, but also drinking and drug problems, depression, undue anxiety and the lack of inner peace.

The actual healing service consisted of three parts:
1. Relaxation and visualisation process
2. Prayers for the sick
3. Laying on of hands and anointing with oil

The reaction of the people was striking and took me by surprise. I have rarely seen people so happy and grateful in church. Tears, of joy, were shed. In the course of the following week a number of cures were reported (although none were investigated or verified).

One lady reported she was cured of a migraine condition from which she had been suffering for a long time. The cure took place at the moment of laying on of hands. Another lady reported a cure from an arthritic hand. For four years she had not been able to open her right hand and at a certain point during the service she noticed the arthritis was not there anymore. A lady who was suffering from very advanced cancer, while not getting an instantaneous cure, found the cancer beginning to recede. Three months later I met her at a subsequent healing service and the recovery, though not yet complete, was still continuing. A family who had heard of the healing service came to participate and to send healing energy to a terminally ill cousin who lived in another part of the United States. That afternoon the family called and informed me that the cousin had undergone a dramatic change about the time of the service, and was well on his way to recovery.

Frank, the parish gardener, a 75 year old Portuguese who had come from the Azores many years before, joined me for a cup of coffee on the morning after the service. I noticed that he was excited. 'Father John', he said, 'I have something very interesting to tell you. I was at your healing service yesterday and something unusual happened. For many years I have suffered from arthritis. Getting up each morning, it takes me about an hour to get my limbs moving. This morning I was on my feet in a matter of minutes. I can't explain it. It seems like a miracle.'

For the first time in my life in the ministry, I realised that there was a real need for healing in the community, a need to be at peace, to be in harmony, a need of which I had been totally unaware, or at least had never thought of in terms of one that would be catered to on a pastoral level.

Now I see healing services as an essential part of the pastoral programme for every community. People need healing all the time. I see the assembled community joined in celebration, in rejoicing, in thanksgiving and in loving, as a powerful healing presence, which generates a 'something', an extraordinarily powerful healing presence, which some people understand in terms of energy, others in terms of grace and others see in terms of the presence of the Holy Spirit.

Subsequently I've conducted a variety of healing services and each one has been an encouraging and enlightening experience. Sometimes the emphasis was on the healing of emotions and other times on the healing of relationships. Wherever the focus was put, that was where the healing took place.

Create Your Own Health Patterns

Children are Natural Healers

When my mother reached her eightieth birthday the family decided to honour the occasion by celebrating Mass in her home. Neighbouring families were present. Children abounded. My niece Ann, a nine month old baby, was suffering from a severe case of whooping cough. Her mother was particularly anxious as two of her own sisters had died in infancy of the illness.

The doctor said Ann was out of danger, but predicted it would be twelve days before she would be really better. During the Mass I suggested we do a healing on the child. I pointed out that the doctor's prediction was probably correct, based on the experience of the medical people, but that we are not limited to the ability of medical science: we have a superior healing power at our disposal. I directed everyone to close their eyes, relax and then send loving vibrations to the child, visualising the child completely well. The children participated with enthusiasm, thrilled by the idea that they could be instrumental in healing Ann. Spiritual authors say that the prayer of children is very powerful, so it was not surprising that thirty minutes later Ann was full of life and vigour.

Carmel

Some six months after my first healing service an elderly man named Paul, who had attended the service, called and asked me if I would pay a visit to his daughter Carmel. She was a fifty-year old lady suffering from advanced cancer. I agreed to visit her but promised no results.

Although still able to move around the house, Carmel spent most of her time lying on the bed, heavily drugged with pain-killers. Her left breast had been removed and she had received radiation therapy on her chest and lower spine. Much burning had taken place and she was in severe pain. On the previous Thursday she had undergone further x-rays, which showed a tumour in the bladder. The doctors had scheduled an operation for the following Monday to remove the tumour.

Since it is my belief that physical sickness is an expression of internal conflict, I began probing to find out if there were any conflicts going on inside of her. No evidence of conflict came to light at that time. Nevertheless I felt that an internal healing was called for – a healing of her emotions. Mine was a simple process, aimed at helping her to let go of any negative feelings such as resentment, envy, fear, guilt or anxiety. I explained to her that all such feelings induce sickness. I encouraged her to see herself in complete peace and harmony with herself and everyone around her.

On this occasion, I also did something which I had not been accustomed to doing when visiting the sick – a laying-on of hands. I recall being distinctly aware of a tremendous energy in my hands.

The following Tuesday morning Paul arrived at my house, very excited. 'Father John,' he said, 'something extraordinary has happened. My daughter was operated on yesterday morning. During the operation she woke up and asked the doctors what they were doing. The doctor answered, 'We can't find your tumour. We have it here on our x-ray charts; we felt it last week during the examination, but it doesn't seem to be here any more!'

A few days later during a subsequent visit she confirmed Paul's story. She felt she had a new lease on life, and although she was still suffering severe pain in her chest and spinal area, she was nevertheless, in a very good disposition, showing much more life than I had seen before. On this occasion I repeated the same healing process concentrating more on her chest and lower back.

During my next visit a week later she confessed that she was having a lot of family problems and was experiencing severe conflict in her life. Her husband was being unfaithful to her, and although she wanted to separate from him, she needed his financial support and insurance to cover her medical expenses. Her daughter would not accept the fact that she continued living with him and, in protest, she left home. Her feeling of isolation and loneliness probably aggravated her illness.

Some days later Carmel had a series of x-rays, and the result came back with the statement: 'There is no evidence of cancer in the body.' Six months later she wrote to me in Brazil saying, 'Thanks be to God I am doing very well.' She also mentioned that she had become reconciled with her daughter.

Regina

The case of Regina is an interesting one. She was fifty years old when her problem began. It was a case of melanoma, a malignant skin cancer. She describes her medical history: 'In April, 1970, I had a birthmark removed from the side of my left leg. It was about the size of an American nickel. It had changed from a brown to a black colour (danger signal!).

'The surgeon said that it was benign. In June, 1973, a lump appeared at the back of my knee and another one at the mid-calf. These were removed through surgical intervention. This time the doctor diagnosed malignancy, but I was not told, though other members of my family knew all about it.

'In November, 1973, I had a further series of tests which showed up another lump on the back of my leg below the calf. This was malignant and once more I had to return to the hospital for major surgery.

'In August, 1974 another lump appeared. It was very small but malignant. It was operated on in September. The doctor cut very deeply and ligaments and tendons were affected. Of all the surgery I had, this left the worst effects.

'In June, 1975 two more lumps appeared, one above the knee and the other almost at the groin. This time the doctors were very worried, as it was the first time the trouble appeared above the knee. These were malignant also. The doctors suggested amputation of the leg, but that really scared me. Eventually they decided on radiation treatment. This went on for six weeks, three times a week.'

It was shortly before this treatment that I got in touch with Regina. She was trying to believe that everything would be all right, but she obviously had a deep anxiety about the outcome. During my visit I tried to stimulate and strengthen her belief in the possibility of healing despite the doctor's negative outlook. I emphasised the importance of desire, positive mental attitudes and belief, as influential factors in the healing process. I also suggested that she do a little probing to see if there were any conflicts, negative feelings or disharmony within her.

Meanwhile through the intermediary of a Japanese friend, I succeeded in getting in touch with a community of Buddhist nuns in Tokyo who had gained renown because of their ability to heal at a distance. Through a process of prolonged meditation they apparently have developed their clairvoyant powers to a very high degree. I asked them what was causing Regina's illness, and what could cure it. A few weeks later a reply came suggesting that the cancer was related to some negative feeling deep within the person. They said, 'Anger, hatred, jealousy, fear and other negative thoughts act on your physical body just like poison and end up taking your own life.' She was instructed to 'reconcile with everything in the universe, especially your parents and ancestors. In the past if you had anger, hatred or jealousy towards someone, meditate and visualise each one with your mind's eye for about ten minutes, while you send out feelings of total forgiveness, and your sickness will disappear'. I was instructed to help draw out all the negative thoughts she may have been keeping in her subconscious, and the sisters promised to keep her in their prayer for three months.

In the course of my next visit, before I told her about the letter or its contents, she took me by surprise by saying, 'You know something, Father? I've been thinking about my sickness a lot. During the week I came to the conclusion that the whole thing is related to a resentment I have been harbouring against certain people who really hurt me some years ago.' Then I handed her the letter. As she read it a look of agreeable surprise showed on her face. That was a turning point for her. From then on whenever I met her and asked her how she was, she invariably answered, 'I am cured. I know I am cured.' In her last letter to me in 1977, she wrote, 'I am 100% well and all I am suffering from is "old age". To prove how well I feel I am back on a full work schedule again. My last visit to the doctor was last month. I had the usual x-rays, etc. All is 100%.'

Kathryn Kuhlman

While working on my thesis I had the opportunity of assisting at a healing service conducted by the internationally known healer, Kathryn Kuhlman.

The service was scheduled for six in the evening, but before ten o'clock people were lining up to get good seats. Some of the 15,000 people who packed the stadium were, like me, curious spectators. Others, more spiritually motivated, were there to share their belief, their prayers and their healing energy with those who needed it. Others had come to be freed from some chronic illness now threatening their very survival. The more severe cases were allotted a central place in the stadium. They were there in hundreds, some on crutches, others on stretchers or in wheel chairs.

This was an ecumenical service, bringing together people and ministers of many creeds. A 2,000 member choir opened the service. Then followed a series of testimonies from people who had been healed after her healing service the previous year. Note, I say 'after' her healing service, because most of those who were healed during the service had an opportunity to give their testimony. Others get their healing as they leave the service, on the way to their cars, on the journey home, or even during the following weeks.

Create Your Own Health Patterns

I recall the testimony of a young man of twenty-four. He had come the previous year in a wheelchair, a victim of cancer. He described the intense pain he had suffered and mentioned that he had lost all his hair from cobalt treatment. He received his healing as he was being helped into the car after the service. Now he was back to give thanks and to give testimony of perfect health. He now had beautiful hair!

The owner of a night club from a town 300 miles away was there, with one of his ex-barmaids. She had been healed of an 'incurable' illness the previous year. As a consequence he had closed his night club and had devoted himself to helping in the healing industry. The testimonies went on.

Then came Kathryn Kuhlman, resplendent in a white dress. In the course of her exhortations she constantly stressed, 'It is not Kathryn Kuhlman who does the healing, but the Holy Spirit'. She seemed to have complete confidence in His power to heal any kind of sickness, and insisted several times that 'all glory must be vowed to the Holy Spirit'.

This went on for almost three hours. Then the scene changed. We were asked to close our eyes, relax and breathe in the Holy Spirit. Then it happened! She felt the healing energy go out from her to someone in the audience. She knew the nature of the illness and the sex of the person at whom it was aimed. She did not know who it was and had only a vague notion of where the person was located. She simply said, 'There is a lady down there getting a healing right now from arthritis. I want you to get up, leave your wheelchair, walk forward and come right up here to the stage. As our eyes searched the stadium, an elderly lady stood up from her wheelchair and slowly moved forward, unsure of her step at first but gaining confidence as she neared the stage. Then she removed a brace which supported her spine and seconds later was running back and forth across the stage, almost totally bewildered by what had taken place.

Then it was a blind man's turn as Kathryn continued,

'There is a man down there receiving a healing from blindness of the left eye. I want you to stand up. Walk forward and come up here to the stage. You can see with both eyes – your sight has been restored'. Seconds later a middle-aged man rose from his seat and made his way forward to the stage.

And so the scene continued for the next hour. The blind had their sight restored, the deaf began to hear again, the crippled left their wheelchairs and walked. Those suffering from heart disease and cancer were instantly cured. It was truly an amazing scene. For me it was a repetition of Jesus' healing.

Kathryn was not satisfied with healing the physical ailment only; she believed inner healing was far more important. In each case she used a ritualistic hand movement on the forehead, followed by an invocation. She called this an 'infusion of the spirit', and apparently this was experienced as an extraordinary sense of peace and harmony.

After the service the many crutches, braces, wheelchairs and stretchers left behind were evidence of a truly amazing happening. I must add, however, that the number cured represented only a small percentage of the total number of sick present.

People wonder how Kathryn Kuhlman became such a powerful healer. What does she have that others don't? I would like to suggest some factors which I believe contributed to her success.

Anyone who studies healing knows the importance of belief in the healing process. It is interesting to note that there was no public propaganda about Kathryn Kuhlman's healings. Instead, groups of believers, such as prayer groups, healing groups, charismatics, pentecostals and small communities, were invited. She eventually succeeded in surrounding herself with a mass of believers, which, when wielded into a community of love must have generated a tremendous energy which became a very powerful healing force. She herself was an exceptionally good channeller, and had enhanced this gift over the years through long daily meditation. Healers say that individual ego needs can absorb healing energy, thus getting in the way of the healing process. Kathryn Kuhlman was constantly removing her ego from the scene by 'vowing all glory to the Holy Spirit'. During the service the singing of the choir induced relaxation and opening up. The individual testimonials, coupled with Kathryn's exhortation, stimulated and enhanced belief. When the time came for the extraordinary to happen, conditions were optimum.

It is often alleged that those healed by Kathryn Kuhlman did not keep their healing. I have met some healed many years ago, and some have kept their health and others have lost it. A relapse may be due to a lack of solid belief on the part of the person healed, or perhaps the belief was dulled by subsequent contact with non-believers. There may also have been a personal need to be ill. Some people cannot live without crutches of one kind or another. Sickness is often an investment. Finally, it may be due to a lack of inner healing. Perhaps inner peace and harmony had not been restored.

The Case of Jack Schwarz

Jack Schwarz, a gifted naturopathic physician and psychic, relates an interesting case of healing, which happened to himself. I quote it because it reinforces my conviction of the need to live in harmony with oneself and with others, of the need to constantly let go of bad feelings, and above all, of the need to forgive.

A resident of the United States, Schwarz was born in Holland, and, like many of his compatriots, was active in the Resistance during the Second World War. Captured by German forces he was transported to a concentration camp. He was tortured in an attempt to extract information. Since he had taught himself voluntary control of internal states he imagined he would be able to endure any degree of physical pain. At a certain point however, he was no longer able to withstand the torture and fainted. While in that state he had a vision of Christ on the cross, and Christ repeated to him the words He addressed to His Father, 'Forgive them, for they know not what they do'. When Schwarz came to, he said to his torturer, 'Ich liebe dich' – I love you. At that point the bleeding stopped and the wounds on his back began healing instantly. The torturer turned pale, threw a sheet over Schwarz and took him to his cell. Schwarz admits that from that day resentment is absent from his life.

Belief and Experience

In this Chapter I have referred to some of the people, the concepts and the experiences which over the years, have served to stimulate my interest and deepen my belief in healing. Had you asked me some years ago if I believed in non-medical healing, I probably would have said 'yes'. But looking back now I realise that my belief was shallow and theoretical.

One's belief is fundamentally based on one's experience and there is a vast difference between a belief based on learned concepts and a belief based on the hard reality of experience. For many years my experience had taught me that when a person contracts a certain ailment he/she goes to the doctors for treatment. If the illness is one that the doctor can normally cure, then the person will get better. If, on the other hand, the illness is one that the doctor cannot normally cure, then the person will not get better.

Today what used to be a shallow belief is now a deep conviction. I have been in touch with people who heal. I have experienced healing myself, and I have witnessed it in other people. Each new healing experience strengthened my belief.

Chapter II

Why Healing Works and Why it Doesn't

*These will be the signs that will be
associated with believers: in my
name they will cast out devils;
they will have the gift of tongues;
They will pick up snakes in their
hands, and be unharmed should they
drink any deadly poison; they will lay
their hands on the sick who will recover.*
MARK 16:17-18

There are many schools of healing, each having its own belief systems and theories, but the same healing phenomena occur in all of them. No one school can claim that because its system works it is the only valid one or that it has all the answers. One's belief then does not have to be built on the absolute truth, but on a rationale related to certain systems of thinking. It can be related to a person, a place, an object or a situation.

For example, many Brazilians believe in spirits. When stricken with bad luck or illness, they ascribe it to the presence of an evil spirit 'closing in' or 'taking possession' of a person or situation. They go to the spiritist centre and by means of a determined ritual, they get rid of, or pacify, the bad spirit. Health and harmony are thus restored.

If one believes in healing by the spirit, such as the Pentecostals, then one's faith will be built on the infinite healing power of the Holy Spirit.

For some it is a belief in a place or an object, such as the grotto at Lourdes, or the relic of a particular saint. For others it is a belief in a special person, such as a particular doctor, a minister, or a healer like Kathryn Kuhlman.

Dona Pachita, world-famous psychic healer in Mexico

City, makes good use of the psychological procedure of involving herself in the clients' thinking systems. With native people she uses herbal treatment, while she prescribes medication for foreigners. In the case of Roman Catholics she often advises them to pray to their favourite saints or get a Mass offered, while Indians are encouraged to make peace with Mother Earth and to carry out some rituals related to nature.

For those who expect a healing accompanied by a ritual she gives a detailed description of how the ritual is to be carried out, in order to ensure the effectiveness of the ceremony. Speaking of psychic surgery she has admitted – and this is quite a confession – it really is not necessary at all, but the operation convinces the patient that something is happening, thus increasing his belief and facilitating the healing.[1]

Recently a friend of mine who spent many years working among the Ibo tribe in Nigeria informed me that the English doctors who went to work with the Ibos had very little success in the application of modern medicine. The reason was they did not have the 'juju' – the magic of the native healing ritual – which was part of the Ibo culture and so necessary for their belief system. The native Ibos who went to England to study medicine and then returned to their own land as qualified medical doctors had a significantly higher degree of success than the non-native doctors. The reason for their success was that they combined medical science with the native juju healing ritual. They healed the body and satisfied the mind.

In his book *The Mind Game: Witchdoctors and Psychiatrists*, E.F. Torrey states, that, 'A witchdoctor who does not share a world view with his patient, does not have personal qualities deemed therapeutic in his culture, cannot raise patient expectation or has no command over therapeutic techniques, will be just as ineffective as the psychiatrist with similar inadequacies.'[2]

Jerome D. Frank contends, 'The apparent success of

healing methods compels the conclusion that the healing power of faith resides in the patients' state of mind, not in the validity of its object.'[3]

Every healer has a system of thought which we may call a philosophy or a world view or a religion, according to which he constructs his healing model and in terms of which he understands and deals with sickness. The successful healer must have the ability to share his thought system with the client in an intelligible manner acceptable to the client, or else must be able to share and understand the thought system of the client.

In other words, he must be capable of offering a rationale to the client which makes sense out of his illness, its causes and its cure. For example, the psychiatrist who tells the illiterate Indian that his phobia is related to oral deprivation will not be understood. Neither will the witchdoctor who tells the American tourist that his sickness is due to possession by a discarnate spirit.[4] Krippner and Villoldo suggest that 'This may be the reason why tourists who show initial improvement following psychic intervention of Dona Pachita or the Filipino spiritists sometimes regress when they return to their homes; their temporary acceptance of the healer's belief system falls apart under the scrutiny of their relatives and neighbours, and so do the benefits they attained'.[5]

Sometimes we find there is a relapse or a recurrence of the illness. This may be due to a lack of complete healing (inner healing) or it may be due to a subsequent weakening of belief.

Our faith can be broken down or weakened by our contact with unbelievers. This is what happened with Bernice, whose case I quoted earlier. Jesus seemed to be aware of this danger also. Many times He warned those He healed to go their way, but to tell no one, implying perhaps, that if you do, people might undermine your faith or 'transmit negative energy'.

Create Your Own Health Patterns

Faith is Fundamental

I believe that one of the basic reasons why more healing does not take place is because people are not tuned into it; they are sceptical about it; they do not really believe it can happen. This lack of faith constitutes an impediment, a resistance to the healing process. Faith is regarded as one of the fundamental conditions for activating the healing process. Faith and healing are so closely linked that when faith in its most general form is not present, healing rarely takes place. Healers are very aware of this and that is why their rituals and ceremonies are designed to stimulate and strengthen the clients' belief. (It would be wrong to conclude that when healing does not take place it is always due to *lack* of faith. It may or may not be. There are various other factors which impede healing.)

Those who believe need to grow in faith. So the quality of one's belief is important. On the part of the healer belief has to be a strong conviction. I have more faith now than I had some years ago. In other words my faith has become stronger and deeper. Consequently, I believe that my healing capacity has improved. This is true of most healers. As they grow in faith and confidence their healing ability becomes more powerful.

On the part of the client, some kind of faith is important. The type of faith I speak of may be simply an implicit belief in, or an awareness of, the possibility of healing. There are various degrees of belief and at its lowest level it may be just an openness to the whole idea of healing.

Writing on this topic Ambrose Worrall states, 'I have an analytical mind and welcome honest scepticism. I think this is good for any type of movement, that all things should be weighed in the balance. Honest scepticism will not prevent the operation of the healing forces because it is not meant as opposition. However, a denial of the possibility that healing can take place is a force that could prevent recovery of a patient'.[6]

Create Your Own Health Patterns

Jesus Demands Faith

Reading through the Gospels one must be impressed by the importance Jesus attached to faith. 'I tell you, therefore, everything you ask and pray for, believe that you have it already and it will be yours,' (Mk 11:24);[7] 'Go in peace, your faith has made you whole' (Mt. 9:22).

He demanded faith from those who wanted healing and so great was His insistence that one gets the impression that without faith He could not help them. Without faith he could not perform His 'works of power'. Many times before healing He asked questions such as 'Do you believe that this is possible?' In the case of the paralysed man, 'My son, your sins are forgiven you. I tell you get up, pick up your mat and go home' (Mk 2: 4-5).

He commended those who had faith. In the case of the woman who touched the hem of His garment in her quest for healing, He greeted her with the remark. 'Courage, my daughter, your faith has made you well' (Mt. 9:22).

When the disciples failed to heal, Jesus rebuked them and attributed their failure to a lack of faith. 'A man came to Jesus, knelt before Him and said to Him, "Sir, have mercy on my son. He is an epileptic and has such terrible fits that he often falls into the fire or water". I brought him to Your disciples, but they could not heal him'. Jesus answered,'How unbelieving and wrong you people are. How long must I stay with you? How long do I have to put up with you? Bring the boy here to me'. Jesus commanded the demon and it went out so that the boy was healed at that very moment. Then the disciples came to Jesus in private and asked Him 'Why didn't we drive the demon out?' And Jesus answered, 'It is because you do not have enough faith' (Mt. 17: 14-20).

Faith is the key which opens the door and releases the healing power. The object of one's faith may vary in accordance with one's philosophical or religious viewpoint. The healing power may be called by different names – grace, Holy Spirit, life energy. They all refer to the same reality which, I believe, is a Divine Presence, which makes whole, integrates and harmonises.

How does faith affect the healing process? Doctor Joseph Murphy attempts to give an explanation. 'The answer to all these healings,' he states, 'is due to the blind belief of the sick person which releases the healing power resident in the subconscious mind.[8] His theory is that universal healing power resides in the subconscious mind and that faith is the process which releases this power for action.

> No mental or religious science practitioner, psychologist, psychiatrist or medical doctor ever healed anybody. There is an old saying 'The doctor dresses the wound but God heals it'. The psychologist or psychiatrist proceeds to remove the mental block in the patient, so that the healing principle may be released, restoring the person to health. Likewise, the surgeon removes the physical block, enabling the healing currents to function normally. No physician, surgeon or mental science practitioner claims that he healed the patient. The one and only healing power is called by many names – nature, God, life, creative intelligence, subconscious power ...
>
> There are many different methods used to remove the mental, emotional or physical blocks which inhibit the flow of the healing life principle animating all of us. The healing principle resident in your subconscious mind can and will, if properly directed by you or someone else, heal your mind and your body of all diseases.[9]

So according to Murphy, the healing power is available, call it whatever name you choose, but the process by which you release it is faith. He also claims that there are many methods or techniques for calling faith into action. The kind of faith he speaks of is a belief that penetrates into the subconscious mind and is accepted by it. The subconscious mind has control of the functions, conditions and sensations of the body and is constantly amenable to the power of suggestion.

Leslie Le Cron in his book *Self Hypnotism* points out that the subconscious is a blind faculty and accepts, without question, whatever the conscious believes, and not only accepts it but acts upon it.[10] It is also a fact that symptoms of almost any disease can be induced in a hypnotic subject by suggestion. For example, a subject in a hypnotic state can develop a high temperature, headache or chest pains, according to the nature of the suggestion given. You can suggest to a person that he is paralysed and cannot walk and it will be so, because the subconscious mind believes it, accepts it as a fact and acts on it.

Harold Sherman, speaking of the place of belief in healing, states;

> In all the centuries that now stretch behind us, a vast multitude of different styles of healing have been performed and most of them have been as successful as the faith invested in them. The healing techniques used, and the rituals, incantations and sacrifices accompanying many of them, do not in themselves possess the power to heal. We know today that any healings that resulted were activated by the power of the mind engendered by faith, which somehow had a restorative effect on the body. To believe constitutes a mighty aid towards recovery, which most members of the medical and psychiatric fraternity will be the first to admit. A person's lack of faith in them and their ministrations makes it much more difficult for them to treat successfully a condition, whether it has been diagnosed as real or imaginary. Faith and spirit healers all stress the power of faith on the part of the patient or subject as a vital and usually necessary adjunct in enabling them to do their healing 'thing'.[11]

Hope and Expectation

Faith and hope are intimately linked. Faith generates hope and hope generates a sense of expectancy which in turn provokes profound changes both in the emotional and psychological state of the person.

Our hopes and desires are such powerful factors that they are capable of determining the course of our lives. We have all heard of people 'dying from a broken heart' at the

Create Your Own Health Patterns

loss of a loved one. Hope and desire disappear. Healers in general have always known that their ability to inspire trust and hope in a patient is a very significant factor for the success of a treatment. Frank points out that assumptions about the future have a very powerful effect on one's present state of mind. A feeling of hopelessness, for example, can impede recovery or even hasten death.[12] In this respect I think it is very important that people in the healing profession refrain from making negative predictions or even negative suggestions regarding the outcome of a certain ailment. Such a prediction, especially when pronounced by a doctor of high repute, is often interpreted by the patient as final and the prediction in time becomes a reality.

On the other hand, as Frank notes, 'mobilisation of hope plays an important part in all types of healing. Favourable expectations generate feelings of optimism, energy, and well-being and may actually promote healing.'[13] This is especially evident in cases of psychosomatic illness. Freud was aware of this, noting that 'expectations coloured by hope and faith are an effective force with which we have to reckon ... in all our attempts at treatment and cure.'[14]

Within the context of hope in relation to healing, I would like to include some reflections on the famous 'Placebo'. The word placebo comes from the Latin and means 'I shall please'. It is defined as 'a substance having no pharmacological effect but given merely to satisfy a patient who supposes it to be a medicine.'[15] It is an inert substance often referred to as a sugar pill, which the doctor administers to a patient to relieve his stress when for one reason or another he does not wish to give an active medicine. The 'placebo effect' can be described as a change in one's state of health, brought about by one's belief or expectancy in relation to a particular object, person, place or situation.

Since the placebo, in the medical sense of the term, is inert, its beneficial effect must lie in its symbolic power. It is generally believed by the medical people today that until a few decades ago most medications prescribed by doctors actually were inert and had no healing power whatever in them. In 1860 Oliver Wendall Holmes stated that if most of the drugs then in use 'could be sent to the bottom of the sea it would be all the better for mankind and all the worse for the fishes.'[16] Shapiro points out in his work *The Placebo Effect in the History of Medical Treatment;* 'The history of medical treatment until relatively recently is the history of the placebo'.[17] In other words, doctors were inadvertently prescribing placebos and getting results.

Over the years a variety of studies and experiments have been made in order to determine more precisely the effect of the placebo and other factors related to it. Frank relates some of these experiments in his book *Persuasion and Healing,* and notes that 'a patient's expectations have been shown to effect his physiological responses so powerfully that they can reverse the pharmological action of a drug.'[18]

In one study of patients hospitalised with bleeding peptic ulcers, 70% showed excellent results lasting over a period of one year, when the doctor gave them injections of distilled water, telling them it was a medicine that would cure them. A control group which received the same injection but were told that it was an experimental medication, showed an improvement of only 25%.[19] The experiment demonstrates that placebo application can activate healing even in the case of severely damaged tissue.

The placebo treatment of warts by painting them with brightly coloured but inert dyes, and telling the patient that the wart will be gone when the dye wears off, is, according to Frank, just as effective as any other form of treatment, (even surgical). It also works on patients who have been unsuccessfully treated by other means. Frank concludes that 'the emotional reaction to a placebo can change the physiology of the skin so that the virus which causes warts can no longer thrive.'[20]

It is also of interest to note that the symbolic meaning of the drug may not always produce favourable results. It is conditioned by the patient's reaction to it. For example, some patients fear certain types of drugs and don't like or perhaps distrust some doctors. In such cases the placebo may produce nausea, diarrhoea or allergies such as skin irritation.[21]

In the psychiatric model we again find ample evidence of the placebo effect response from the patient. Prompt symptomatic relief is a frequent occurrence following the initial contact with the psychiatrist. Various studies have suggested that this is due to the patient's high degree of expectancy.

With regard to the frequency of visits to the psychiatrist, it has been noted that when psychoanalysis was introduced to America from Europe, the clients going only once or twice a week for one year in the States got the same results as those going five or six times a week for a year in Europe. The reduction did not depend on the severity of the illness.[22] It seems that the hopes both of the doctors and the psychiatrist are transmitted to the patient and to a certain degree his response is conditioned by them.

Experiments with placebos lead one to the conclusion that the hope of the patient is a very important factor in recovery. Speaking of this, Frank states 'The intensity of hope that can be elicited by psychotherapy must be a pale shadow of that evoked by religious healing.[23]

The Question of Lourdes

Though the Catholic Church is not in the forefront in the healing world, nevertheless, down through the ages, it at least has been open to the idea of healing through divine intervention. Today the shrine of Lourdes has become world famous as a place of pilgrimage and has become of particular interest in the western Christian world because of the many cures deemed to have taken place there.

Although the Church believes in miracles, nevertheless, it stipulates that only when all the possible 'natural' explanations have been exhausted may we resort to an explanation of a 'supernatural' nature for a given occurrence. It lays

Create Your Own Health Patterns

down the most demanding criteria which must be fulfilled before a given case is pronounced a miraculous cure. For example, in order that a cure at Lourdes be regarded as miraculous, it must be a healing from a disease pronounced incurable by the medical profession. The person healed must have undergone a battery of tests before the healing takes place and another battery of tests after it has occurred. Complete documentation is required.

Soon after Bernadette Soubirous experienced her famous visions in 1858 some miraculous cures were reported. The number of pilgrims to Lourdes has steadily increased over the years, and today over two million visit the grotto annually, including some thirty thousand sick. To date only sixty-two cases have passed the stringent test required by the Catholic Church in order to be considered miraculous. Of course many more healings or partial healings have taken place, but have not been pronounced miracles due to lack of proper documentation.

I would like to note here that a healing does not have to be miraculous, or even a complete cure, in order to be considered a healing. Any significant improvement in one's health, though not a complete cure, signifies healing, and many healings of this nature happen at Lourdes. Yet the total number of healings which have taken place at Lourdes represent a very small fraction of the sick who have made the pilgrimage.

Although the Church has pronounced some cures at Lourdes as being miraculous, many psychologists would understand them as phenomena brought about by a psychological process. Some would hold that the healing which occurs is the result of the patient's response to an increase in faith and a building up of new hope through an experience which is highly emotional.

Frank gives a vivid description of the typical pilgrims experience in Lourdes and in his analysis of it, he draws attention to certain factors which, in his own opinion, make it a highly emotional experience. Those who go to Lourdes are

Create Your Own Health Patterns

usually chronic cases who have failed to respond to medical treatment. They have become isolated in their community, have come to regard themselves as burdens to others, and have a very bleak outlook on the future. The decision to go to Lourdes changes all this. The patient once more becomes the centre of attention and breaks through his isolation and routine. Funds are collected, medical examinations are carried out, and travel arrangements are made. Not only the family members but the community at large is involved in the process. Prayers, Masses and Novenas are offered for the success of the pilgrimage. One's faith is also stimulated by the attitude of other pilgrims.[24] Frank suggests that the 'emotional excitement connected with the preparatory period and the journey to the shrine may be essential for healing to occur.'[25]

On arrival at Lourdes the pilgrim's hopes are further enhanced. He is plunged into a city of pilgrims, coming from the four corners of the earth seeking one thing, a healing for themselves and their loved ones. Everyone hopes to witness or experience a miraculous cure. Previous cures are recounted. The piles of discarded crutches are witness to previous healings.[26]

There are three high points in the pilgrimage which have a great emotional impact on the sick; the immersion in the ice-cold spring, the procession climaxing the days' activities and the reception of Holy Communion. After careful scrutiny of the whole process Frank suggests that the cures in Lourdes are not miraculous but rather the result of a process activated by an intense emotional impact. He notes, 'It is interesting in this connection that, except for original cures, Lourdes has failed to heal those who live in its vicinity.'[27]

Some cures occur en route to Lourdes, others on the way home, and others still weeks or months later. The type of people cured are 'almost invariably simple people – the poor and the humble; people who do not interpose a strong intellect between themselves and the High Power'.[28] It is generally agreed that people who remain emotionally unmoved by what goes on do not experience cures. All this lends support to Frank's arguments. If his theory on Lourdes is valid then the same kind of analysis can be applied to other healing shrines such as Fatima in Portugal, Guadalupe in Mexico, Knock in Ireland and Aparecida do Norte in Brazil.

It is important to note that inexplicable cures of serious or organic diseases occur quite frequently in medical practice. Many doctors can testify to cases of patients mysteriously recovering from seemingly fatal illness. Two surgeons have assembled data on 176 cases of cancer which regressed without 'proper' medical treatments.[29] If such cases occurred at Lourdes they might be spoken of in terms of miracles. How one understands them really depends on one's framework of thinking.

Many controversies have taken place over the authenticity and the miraculous nature of cures which have taken place at Lourdes and elsewhere. But, as Frank points out, many of these controversies have to be based on the erroneous assumption that one's rejection of the miraculous nature of the healings implies a rejection of miracles as such, or of a doctrine of the Catholic Church.[30]

It is actually quite feasible to accept some Lourdes cures as authentic while maintaining scepticism about their miraculous cause. Furthermore it is possible to be a devout and authentic Catholic while rejecting modern miracles.[31]

Wrong Mental Attitudes

If we can get to the point of accepting the idea that we are responsible for most of our illnesses, then we also become responsible for the healing of those same illnesses and can facilitate the process enormously by our mental attitudes and emotional input.

Our contemporary society in general is not tuned into belief in non-medical healing. We are medically conditioned, and this is so deep-rooted in us that we offer enormous resistance to accepting a different concept of healing or an alternate healing approach. Only fifty years ago the French psychotherapist, Emile Coue, who established his own private hospital at Nancy, was having great success in the treatment of all types of ailments, despite the fact that medication was never applied.[32]

Coue always stressed that he was not primarily a healer but one who taught people to heal themselves. His formula 'Every day and in every way I am getting better and better', which his patients recited several times a day, has become famous. His teachings at the time spread rapidly and he drew enormous crowds, not only to his hospital in France but also to his lectures in England and the United States.

With subsequent progress in medical science and especially with the development of antibiotics, the tide began to turn in favour of a more sophisticated, official type, of medicine which apparently began to give immediate results. This rapid development in medicine, coupled with the economic and social pressures behind it, became one important factor in weaning the western mind away from non-medical healing.

Sickness for us is a kind of 'mystery'. We have no clear ideas of where it comes from, what its presence means, nor what should be our attitude towards it. Almost all of us are contaminated by erroneous mental attitudes, inherited from our family, religious and cultural backgrounds.

Does God Send Sickness?

One such attitude is that God sends sickness. Of course such a mentality completely undermines belief in non-medical healing, especially in healing through prayer. Behind this idea is the notion proposed by Christian teachings that sickness is the result of original sin and since everyone is born with original sin, sickness is part of man's destiny.

Another attitude is the belief that God, though not sending illness directly, nevertheless allows it to happen for some specific purpose. This is known as the 'permissive will' of

Create Your Own Health Patterns

God. The underlying belief is that God permits the illness for some reason unknown to us and our attitude should be one of acceptance with resignation.

These attitudes give rise to doubt, confusion and conflict within the person. If I am in doubt as to whether my illness is God's will or not, and I am praying for recovery, my prayer, no matter how fervent will reflect that doubt, which is deeply embedded in my mind and probably will impede the healing process. Francis MacNutt in his book *Healing* points out that 'Our attitude toward sickness, whether to ask God to remove it, or to accept it as his will,' becomes a key issue in healing.[33]

Everything that happens to us in life is not necessarily God's will and sickness certainly is not. The attitude 'May God's will be done' can easily engender a fatalistic mentality in face of life's problems and especially in relation to sickness.

I have often heard people say that 'sickness brings one closer to God'. Sometimes it does and sometimes it does not. While admitting that it does, I believe one does not have to become ill in order to get close to God.

Some people believe that suffering in the form of illness is a sign of God's special favour. God visits his loved ones with sickness and invites them to carry their cross as loyal disciples of Jesus. This is a message commonly conveyed to sick people by spiritual preachers and hospital chaplains in their efforts to console and strengthen them. It is a confusing message to which people react differently. Some may say, 'Perhaps in asking God to take away my sickness I am refusing to carry my cross', while others may ask, 'If God is good why does he allow this to happen to me'. This a very common reaction in Brazil and sometimes leads to a total rejection of God.

MacNutt states that, 'Undue emphasis on the cross and the benefits of suffering has been a factor in displacing both the belief in and the desire for healing among many Christians'. The suffering that Christ promised His followers was not the suffering of sickness but rather the consequences of living out His Christian message – the rejection, the alienation, the hate, the torture, the self sacrifice. Suffering is part of everybody's life, but not necessarily in the form of sickness. Jesus experienced much more suffering than the normal human person, but I doubt if sickness was part of it.

As a healer Jesus is a very interesting study, not only because of the marvellous works he performed, but also because of His whole attitude towards illness which stands in sharp contrast to the attitude of most Christians today.

He regarded sickness as an evil (contrary to the popular view of the time that sickness was a punishment from God) and His attitude toward disease was one of disdain and scorn. Nowhere in the Bible is it recorded that He refused to heal. On the contrary it is said 'He healed everybody'. He did say that in his own home town of Nazareth He was unable to perform any 'works of power' because of a lack of faith on the part of the inhabitants; 'and He did not work any miracles there because of their lack of faith' (Mt. 13:58).

The Importance of Desire

A real desire to get well has to be present for healing to take place. Here again the attitude of Jesus is interesting. Rather than go out and offer His services to heal the sick He seemed to wait for the sick to come to him and solicit His help. This is evident in such petitions as 'Please help her', 'Lord, if You wish You may make me clean', 'Jesus, son of David, have pity on me'. In fact He sometimes demanded explicit evidence of this desire on the part of the sick. In the case of the blind beggar Bartimaeus, Jesus said to him, 'What do you want Me to do for you?' And the blind man said, 'Master, that I may see' (Mk 10:51).

Doctors are the first to admit that a patient has to have a desire to get well in order that normal recuperation takes place. Despite all their skills and learning they sometimes find themselves helpless in the presence of a patient who lacks the desire.

Psychologists and counsellors put much emphasis on the importance of the client's motivation as a condition for the successful outcome of therapy. Motivation in this sense is understood as a desire to be in therapy because one hopes to achieve real benefit from it.

Alcoholics Anonymous knows full well that in order for the alcoholic to quit his drinking habit, he must first of all recognise that he has a problem, admit that he needs help and express his desire to recuperate by attending the meetings.

In his book *Man's Search for Meaning*,[34] Viktor Frankl describes his three years in a German concentration camp during the Second World War. He attributes his survival, not to the chance circumstance of his being one of the lucky ones, but to his 'will to leave', his own deep desire to survive because he had a purpose in life, something in life he wanted to achieve.

Some healings do not take place because there is a lack of real desire to get well. The same is probably true in many instances where there is a relapse. Sickness can be an investment for some people. It has its compensations attached to it. In some cases the patient may need to be ill in order to survive in the structure into which he has put himself. 'What will I do now that my sickness is gone? I can't live without it.'

I recall one day visiting a lady in her sixties who was ill in bed. Though she looked quite healthy, she had already had several serious ailments, including two strokes. She was very lonely and complained about everything. Her bedroom resembled a drugstore, she had such a variety of medication. After conversing with her for a little while, I came to the conclusion that in her present state of mind, neither God nor man could cure her. She needed to be ill, for that was the only way she got attention, even though she got most of it from herself.

Need to Find a Specific Cause

Some spiritual healers seem to get better results when they specify the type of healing. This is especially the case in the healing of emotional scars, and harmful memories. Here, of course, an understanding of psychology is a definite advantage. This is a very interesting factor and MacNutt gives a lot of importance to it, stating that 'Several times I have prayed for inner healing, knowing we were praying about the right problem, and yet nothing happened. It was only when we went back and found the root incident, which had been forgotten, and then performed the healing service, that the healing actually took place.'[35]

He quotes the case of the leader of a healing group who wanted to quit smoking. His group prayed for him to give up the bad habit while another group prayed for his deliverance, but he continued to smoke and no matter how hard he tried he just could not succeed in quitting. Some months later, hearing a talk on inner healing, he realised that his smoking habit was related to his teen years when smoking represented to him freedom and adulthood. In particular, it represented the freedom he needed from the overcontrolling authority of his father. The key to his being free from the smoking habit was connected to his need for inner healing. So in a subsequent session when the group prayed for a healing of his relationship with his father, he quit his smoking habit.[36]

In the field of psychology various approaches are used in order to get to the specific root of problems. A psychoanalyst can spend months and sometimes years working with one client trying to get to the specific cause of a disturbance. Some therapists use age-regression as a technique to get in touch with certain traumatic experiences which are no longer available to the conscious mind. This process is often essential in order to effect a complete healing. Like good doctors and good psychiatrists, the good healer needs to discern what is the hidden cause behind those symptoms.

Create Your Own Health Patterns

Salvation Means Wholeness

Plato's dualism – seeing the human person's make-up as two separate principles, soul and body – heavily influenced the Stoics, the Manicheans, the Cartesians and finally the Jansenists. Traditionally in our Christian culture we have retained this dualistic concept of man. The salvation of Christ has been understood in terms of the saving of the soul and the church's missionary activity traditionally has been referred to in terms of 'saving souls'. Since the soul was understood as the permanent principle, the immortal part of man, the salvation of the soul became the all important purpose of life, with almost total disregard for the body.

In Hebrew thinking, man was never conceived of in terms of body and soul but as a whole person, and healing meant not saving souls but healing the person.

Modern psychology has helped to put man together again and tends to treat man not as body and soul but as a person. Even some modern theologians speak of salvation in terms of the liberation of the whole person. Speaking in this context, Bishop Helder Camera of Recife, Brazil says, 'I have never met a soul during my whole life, but I have met very many people.'

Although the dualistic concept of the person has been officially condemned by the church, nevertheless it is still very evident not only in the language used by the church, but also in some of its pastoral practices. A typical example of this is the traditional use of the sacrament of Anointing in the Roman Catholic church (See Chapter One). The scriptural basis for this sacrament is found in the Epistle of St James: 'Is there anyone who is sick? He should call the church elders, who will pray for him and rub oil on him in the name of the Lord. This prayer made in faith will heal the sick man; the Lord will restore him to health and the sins he has committed will be forgiven' (Js 5: 14-15). It seems clear from this text that the anointing with oil is intended primarily to heal the sick person from illness. Yet, in practice, the Catholic church has used this sacrament for centuries as a means of forgiving sin and preparing the sick person for death. It has even been called the sacrament of Extreme Unction or the Last Anointing, and its very use has been restricted to those in danger of death from sickness.

In recent times, however, there has been a change in thinking regarding the anointing of the sick and the actual name has been changed to the sacrament of Anointing or the sacrament of Healing.

Jesus Proclaims His Healing Mission

I have read the Gospel accounts of Jesus' life many times and as I re-read them I am impressed by the importance Jesus gave to the healing ministry and the amount of time he devoted to it. His healing ministry was an integral part of his salvation process. His message of salvation was not one of saving souls, but of liberating man from all those forces that oppress him, that keep him in bondage and cause him suffering. One of those forces is disease. Jesus was concerned with saving the whole man and healing was part of it. 'The Spirit of the Lord has been given to me, for he has anointed me. He has sent me to bring the good news to the poor, to proclaim liberty to the captives, to bring sight to the blind, to set the downtrodden free and to proclaim the Lord's favour' (Lk. 4: 18-19).

Jesus obviously saw His salvation as applied to the whole person and that is why He was so concerned about the body. His message of salvation was one of liberation, of healing and of wholeness. As MacNutt states, 'Healing is simply the practical application of the basic message of salvation, a belief that Jesus wanted to liberate us from personal sin and from emotional and physical illness.'[37]

Anybody Can Do It

Today many people see Jesus as an outstanding psychic en-

Create Your Own Health Patterns

dowed with highly developed abilities. For some His extraordinary performances were not miraculous phenomena but the result of normal abilities inherent in every human being.

MacNutt notes that Jesus did not stress the miraculous but the ordinary nature of His healing ministry. He referred to His achievements not as miracles but as works of power. 'They were, so to speak, the normal thing for him to do. They formed an integral part of His mission'.[38] Jesus commanded His apostles to preach, teach and heal the sick. 'He called the twelve together and gave them power and authority over all devils and to cure all diseases and He sent them out to proclaim the Kingdom of God and to heal the sick' (Lk. 9: 1-2).

The command was extended not only to the twelve apostles but to all His disciples: 'After this Jesus appointed seventy-two others and sent them out ahead of Him in pairs to all the towns and places He Himself was to visit' (Lk. 10:1). 'Whenever you go into a town where they make you welcome, eat what is put before you. Cure those in it who are sick and say, "The Kingdom of God is at hand"' (Lk. 10:8-9). Later there is mention of the joyous return of the seventy-two and how they jubilantly related their success to Jesus. 'Lord,' they said, 'even the demons obeyed us when we commanded them in Your name' (Lk. 10: 17).

Healing was an integral part of the ministry in the early church. In the Acts of the Apostles we find many references to healing performed not only by the original apostles but also by Paul and various other followers of Jesus who did not belong to the original twelve. For them healing seemed to be a very normal procedure.

Finally, according to the Gospel of Mark, all believers have a share in the healing ministry. 'Go out to the whole world, proclaim the good news to all creation. And these will be the signs that will be associated with believers; in My name they will cast out devils; they will have the gift of tongues; they will pick up snakes in their hands, and be unharmed if they drink any deadly poison; they will lay

Create Your Own Health Patterns

their hands on the sick, who will recover' (Mk 16: 17-18).

Now the big question is, if Jesus laid so much importance on healing and was insistent that His apostles and disciples heal the sick, why is it that the Catholic church and other Christian churches today give so little importance to the Master's injunction?

Chapter III

Energy Transference and Healing

People tormented by unclean spirits were also cured, and everyone in the crowd was trying to touch Him because power came out of Him that cured them all.
LUKE 6:19

The term 'energy' has become a much used word in the vocabulary of people in the healing profession. Many of those involved in healing understand the operation in terms of a transference of energy, from the healer to the person being healed.

Wilhelm Reich is the great modern exponent of the energy theory. When he developed his orgone box he saw it as a means of accumulating orgone energy in concentrated form, and hoped, through this, to cure illness, including cancer. At a certain point in the development of his energy some of his followers thought he had gone insane. Yet today he has gained a lot of credibility and many contemporary thinkers are influenced and stimulated by some of his concepts of energy.

Many present day healers understand the process in terms of the transference of energy. They speak of re-charging one's energy, of feeling energy, of measuring energy and of letting the energy flow. This whole question of energy has become the object of much discussion. Laboratory experiments being carried out point to interesting conclusions.

Some experiments were conducted by Sister Justa Smith, a biochemist and enzymologist, in conjunction with 'Mr E', a seventy-six year old retired Hungarian army colonel who had highly developed healing power. In the laboratory this healing power was directed towards wounded mice, dis-

Create Your Own Health Patterns

tressed barley seedlings and depressed enzymes.[1]

Other experiments were conducted by Bernard Grad, a young biochemist from McGill University. In one of these experiments numerous mice were wounded in the laboratory in identical fashion and treated in one of three ways: by Mr E, by an 'ordinary' individual or by nothing at all. The mice treated by Mr E healed at significantly higher rates than those in the other two groups. In another experiment conducted by Grad it was discovered that seedlings nourished with water that Mr E had merely held in his hands grew more vigorously than those nourished by untreated water.

Smith, in her experiment with Mr E decided to use an enzyme called trypsin. It is her theory that since enzymes are necessary for catalysing all metabolic reactions within cells, all bodily malfunctions will manifest themselves to some extent at the enzyme level. Thus if the body is to be healed of some malfunction, the healing process must also manifest itself at the enzyme level.

During the initial experiment – which lasted three weeks under scientifically controlled conditions – Mr E consistently increased the activity of depressed enzymes, to a statistically significant degree, by the laying on of hands. The enzymes not treated by him did not regain activity. The same experiments with people not professed to have healing power effected no change in the enzymes. Smith concluded that there must have been a transference of energy but could not determine what kind of energy it was.

An interesting factor showed up in the next series of experiments in the next year. Mr E had no influence whatever on the enzymes.

This may be explained by the fact that during the previous experiment it was vacation time with no activity on campus and Mr E was happy and tranquil. On the second visit, however, Mr E was upset both by a personal problem and by the activity on the campus. Smith concluded that the ability of the healer depends on his personal state of mind.

Create Your Own Health Patterns

In yet another experiment carried out on wounded mice, a statistical analysis showed that wounds of the animals treated by Mr E healed faster then those of any other group. Mice treated by sceptical medical students healed more slowly then mice that received no laying on of hands at all.

Speaking of the experiments, Dr Grad states, 'Although little can be said about the nature of the force that is producing the biological effects ... or the mechanism whereby it acts, the experiments on wound healing and plant growth have demonstrated that the so-called laying on of hands, at least when done by certain individuals, has objective effects ... which can hardly be explained as due to the power of suggestion. It seems apparent that to the extent that suggestion is effective, it is itself an energy.'[2]

Smith also came to the conclusion that one cannot say that the healing process is psychosomatic, that it is due to the power of suggestion nor that it is in your head: 'Enzymes don't have heads.'

Besides his laboratory work, Mr E had some very interesting healings on humans and animals. Once he healed his twelve year old son simply by holding him for days. He himself attributed this healing to what he called a 'parent's love'. It has also been observed that while he was in the military the horses he rode never tired.

Speaking of actual healing process Mr E confessed he did not know what happened but believed an energy passed from him to the patient.

In January 1975 a research team composed of Dr Robert N. Miller, an industrial research scientist, and Dr Philip B. Reinhart, head of the physics department of Agnes Scott College, and student assistant Anita Kern conducted some experiments with the internationally known healer Olga Worrall at Agnes Scott College near Atlanta, Georgia.[3] The key experiment had the objective of determining whether or not some type of measurable energy is given off the healer's hands.

The detection device was an Atomic Laboratories Model

71850 cloud chamber. When members of the investigating teams placed their hands around the cloud chamber to see if they could influence the cloud pattern, there was no discernible effect. When Worrall performed, placing her hands at the side of the chamber without touching the glass while visualising energy flowing from her hands (much as she does when treating a patient), the observers saw a definite wave pattern develop in the cloud. When Worrall shifted her position 90 degrees to see if the wave pattern would be effected, the waves actually changed direction, and began moving perpendicularly to the original path.

On 12 March 1974 an experiment was carried out to see if Worrall could effect the cloud chamber from a distance. This time the cloud chamber stayed in Atlanta. Worrall was in Baltimore, 600 miles away. She was asked to repeat what she had actually done in the previous experiments. During the time of her concentration a definite change took place in the cloud chamber – a kind of turbulence. The turbulence continued for some minutes after Worrall had finished her process. When asked about this later she suggested that the cloud chamber had become charged with some type of energy and a certain amount of time was necessary for its dissipation. She also added that in local and distant healing the energy acts much as it did in the cloud chamber; it churns up activity and stimulates cell action.

By way of conclusion, the research team suggested that the experiment lends support to the theory that a tangible energy issues from the hands of healers when mentally directed. The results of the second experiment indicate that 'thoughts are things', and visible manifestations in the physical world can be produced mentally from a distance.

Laboratory experiments do seem to indicate that there is a definite transference of energy during healing. Many questions have still got to be answered. Of what does this energy consist? How is it transferred? What part does the imagination play? Does belief have anything to do with ability to transfer it?

Create Your Own Health Patterns

Transmission of Energy

Many healers, both spiritual and psychic, who operate through the laying on of hands, understand the process that takes place in terms of a transmission of energy from the healer to the person being healed. But the energy they speak of is not a physical energy nor is it a psychological energy derived from a state of well-being of the healthy person. The healers claim that there exist other types of energies which they call 'life energies'. These can be tapped and utilised.

According to Olga Worrall, her healing involves channelling of energy into the healee. This energy comes from what she refers to as a 'universal field of energy' which is common to all creation. She understands it as ultimately coming from God, the source of all power. She speaks of 'emanations' that surround the individual, caused by 'electrical currents' which can be seen as auras by people with psychic abilities. She also speaks of 'sound waves' emanating from the various physical organs, 'thought waves' from the mind and 'vibration' from the spiritual body. The healer, by tuning in his or her personal energy field to the universal field of energy and making contact with universal energy, acts as a type of conductor between it and the person being healed.[4] (This reminds me of the concept of the operation of grace, as understood by the traditional Catholic theology.)

Speaking of her husband, who is also a healer, Worrall stated, 'Of course Ambrose as a scientist has always made sense of this explanation. He says that spiritual healing is a rearrangement of the microparticles of which all things are composed. The body is not what it seems to be with the naked eye. It is not a solid mass. It is actually a system of little particles or points of energy, separated from each other by space and held in place through an electrically balanced field. When these particles are not in their proper places then disease is manifested in the body. Spiritual healing is the process which re-establishes those particles in harmonious relationships – which means good health.'[5]

Create Your Own Health Patterns

Worrall refers to herself as a spiritual healer rather than a psychic healer because according to her, such psychic abilities as telepathy and clairvoyance are not necessarily involved with the phenomena. She goes on to state, 'The spiritual healing I do is enhanced by my psychic gift but spiritual healing can be and usually is accomplished by people who are neither clairvoyant, clairaudient, nor mediumistic in any way. The healing current flows through every clear channel available, whatever the healer's psychic abilities, or, for that matter, religious belief.' She insists there are no guaranteed healings, and that she does not do the healing; 'The spiritual power comes from God; I put my hands on someone and pray but it is God who does the healing.'[6]

The Human Aura

Not only humans, but animals, plants and even inanimate matter give off a certain emanation and are surrounded by energy fields in a three dimensional level. These energy fields are called by various names, the most common one being the 'aura'. According to those who have made a detailed study of the topic, the human aura can be seen in the form of a series of energy fields surrounding the human body. Jack Schwarz distinguishes seven in all and he refers to them as the 'seven auric fields'.[7] The energy fields can change in size, density and colour, in response to physiological, emotional, mental or spiritual changes in the human person.

The first energy field, which is the most visible, surrounds the whole body, accompanying all its contours. It is the one closest to the physical body and has been referred to by the esoteric writers as the 'etheric body'. Jack Schwarz calls it the 'Physical Aura'.[8] It is a kind of extension of the physical body and is, in fact, susceptible to touch. In other words the human person extends away further than the skin. It is a common experience to feel goose pimples on one's skin when certain persons get close to us. In fact, we can sometimes feel the proximity of another person without using any of the five senses and at times we even have difficulty in distinguishing between the proximity and the touch. This is due to the physical aura which in certain cases can extend up to twelve inches from the body. This aura seems to be closely related to the physiological part of the person and can be used to diagnose physical ailments by those who know how to read and interpret it.

Outside of the physical aura there exists a series of other energy fields, each one reflecting a specific aspect of the human person. They are similar to the physical aura in that they are made up of the same electromagnetic particles, but they differ from it in that they are composed of a much finer and more subtle substance. Nor do they follow the contours of the body like the physical aura but can be seen in the shape of an egg surrounding the human body. The aura presents a very faithful picture of the person. It reflects not only the physical and emotional state of the person, but also the degree of one's mental and spiritual development.

The aura exists as a vital force, but in general, we don't succeed in seeing it. Because of our lack of visual sensitivity we have lost touch with it. In recent times a variety of instruments and techniques have been developed to help us to see the aura more clearly. Presently a lot of research is being done on the topic. There is some hope of developing a process whereby the human can be photographed and the photograph used for diagnosing illness. The most famous of these experiments to date is the well known Kirlian photography. This technique developed by a Russian, Seymon Kirlian, is aimed at photographing the aura of animals and plants. In general people believe they cannot see the human aura, but in fact it is clearly visible to psychics. Artists depicting saints or mystics often represent them surrounded by auras. Children in general have more facility than adults in seeing the aura. They often observe it around their parents or teachers and are sometimes scoffed at when they relate their visions to their elders. Those under the influence of alcohol or other drugs can be quite adept at seeing auras. In fact, with a little training, most people are capable of observing auras. In his book *Human Energy System*,[9] Schwarz describes in detail a number of eye exercises aimed at facilitating this process.

Sickness is understood as static energy and energy particles gone astray, and is reflected in the human aura. The laying on of hands is nothing more than a charge transmitted from the healer to get the energy in motion again, or to get the particles back in the right order.

Olga Morrall uses aura reading for diagnostic purposes and seems to be able to recognise an ailment from the colours and size of the aura. During her laying on of hands some observers have noticed an 'almost colourless thin kind of vapoury stuff that floats like smoke from the space between her hands and the healer's body.'[10] When asked what she feels during the operation she replied, 'When I put my hands on a person a heat seems to be generated from my hands. People say it feels like hot pads. Sometimes I experience a sensation, like an electrical discharge, with pins and needles pricking on my palms and fingertips.'[11] Many healers know when they are in contact; they feel the energy go out from them. Jesus said He felt 'virtue' going out of Him when He healed.

A Psychic Healing

At the time I was working on my thesis, I made a visit to a psychic healing group at the Inner Light Foundation of Novato, California. My official purpose in going there was research, so I was allowed to participate with the group in the whole healing process, and also experience a personal healing. I had been feeling a lot of anxiety, which I attributed to being behind in my work. I was also suffering from stomach pains but for some strange reason I did not mention this fact to the group.

The session began with a prolonged meditation. A brief

meditation was then made before working on each client. When my turn came I was instructed to lie on a couch, close my eyes and relax. The group sat around me, one member at my head, one at my feet and one on either side, with hands extended towards me but not touching my body. Sam, on my left – who was said to have powerful energy – held his left hand raised in a vertical position (as a kind of antenna) while he extended his right hand in my direction.

Olivia, on my right, repeated a number of hand passes over me. Jerome at my feet was the psychic in the group, and he told me privately what images he had picked up during the process, and incidentally asked me if I was having any stomach trouble. During the process I felt a tremendous sensation of heat all over my body, and my hands particularly were vibrating with a warm energy. The group assured me that my work would be very successful and that I would have no further anxiety about it. From that time my work actually began to run more smoothly. There was a reduction in anxiety, and the stomach pains disappeared. Of course, I have no way of verifying if this was due to the transmission of healing, a renewal of hope or some other factor.

Laying on of Hands and the Aura

Back in the eighteenth century the famous controversial healer Franz Anton Mesmer developed a healing procedure which combined 'laying on of hands', 'exorcism' and transmitting energy through an 'electric fluid'. He also spoke of the aura or energy body surrounding the human body. According to him, sickness in the physical body expresses itself in the aura in the form of an energy imbalance. In his thinking the physical body takes its healing from the energy body. By working on the energy body, physical healing takes place. This can be done in two ways; one, by manipulating the energy with hand movements (laying on of hands) and two, by the use of the imagination. He conceived of this energy as being under the control of the imagination and

Create Your Own Health Patterns

consequently capable of being manipulated by it.

Allan Kardec followed the line of Mesmer, believing 'that the "spirit" is enveloped in a semi-material body of its own which he names "peri spirit". This peri spirit is composed of magnetic fluid which contains a certain amount of electricity. It serves as an intermediary between one's "spiritual body" and physical body.' Thus Kardec stated that healing can be accomplished by psychic healers who send 'magnetic rays' from their fingertips into the 'aura' of ill persons. By using these 'magnetic passes' a healer can also magnetise water which can be used for healing purposes.[12] Today in Brazil many spiritist mediums who follow the line of Kardec use the aura for diagnostic purposes and apply the laying on of hands or hand passes as a healing technique.

Becoming a Clear Conduit

Does one's healing energy get drained? If so, how does one conserve it or recharge it? When asked about this Olga Worrall replied, 'Why should I get tired or my energy get drained? The energy is not mine. It comes from a superior universal source.'[13]

The important questions are how to get in touch with this universal or cosmic energy and how to become a good conduit and let it flow.

Yoga and Energy

Many of the yoga practices work toward 'purifying and activating' the seven chakras, or energy centres of the human body. Adepts speak of the 'Kundalini' energy, or 'serpent power', which resides at the base of the spine, like a coiled serpent waiting to rise. When the Kundalini energy has risen through all seven chakras one is said to have become an 'initiate' and is regarded as having gained master control of mind and body, and well on the path to cosmic knowledge. Carl Jung spoke of the sublimation of this energy through the energy centres by the practice of yoga.

Pierre Weil in his book *A Conscienda Cosmica* states: 'This energy is located in a sexual centre called *Mulhadra*, from where the 'Kundalini' (the name given to it which is symbolised by a serpent) rises through the vertical column, until at a level just above the head it meets the cosmic energy which comes down from space, thus achieving the cosmic union of Shiva and Shakti.'[14] Teilhard de Chardin states that one of the principal functions of man is the transformation and the propagation of universal energy. Yoga and meditation are understood as systems which help to achieve this. Other practices or disciplines such as celibacy, fasting and isolation are also seen as aids towards achieving the same goal.

Celibacy

Some schools of thought maintain that those who practice celibacy are more effective healers.

Many of the great saints and mystics of the Catholic tradition practised total abstinence from sexual activity. Moses asked his followers to observe three days of abstinence from sexual activity before promulgating the ten commandments. For many of the famous yogis, abstinence from sexual activity is regarded as a very fundamental discipline for growth on the path of initiation. In the spiritual traditions of Brazil, healers and mediums are recommended to abstain from sexual relations on the day they work in the centre.

For some months I was associated with a yoga community in San Francisco. It was a mixed community of males and females, all celibate. When I asked them what importance celibacy had in their lifestyle, I was told, 'It has something to do with making energy available for other purposes.'

On the other hand, some maintain that sexual relations with the right partner in a fulfilling and life-giving experience in no way depleted energy but actually facilitates its

Fasting

Fasting is another discipline that is recommended as an aid towards spiritual development. It has been a very strong tradition in Christian religious communities particularly in the Catholic church. Unfortunately it has been seen primarily as a mere ascetic discipline without any clear understanding of the real purpose and value of it. Most yoga traditions practice fasting. Some abstain from certain foods such as meat and eggs; others do prescribed periods of fasting from all food.

I have spoken to a number of people who have done research on fasting and have been through fasting experiences themselves and they all agree on certain basics. In our society we tend to over-eat and consume certain foods that not only do not provide the type of nourishment we need, but are positively harmful to our health. In our culture obesity has become a common problem. One very sure way of dealing with it is fasting.

The experts also tell us that periodic fasting not only detoxifies the body, but also tones up the senses, clarifies the mind and facilitates our spiritual development.

Most of us are familiar with stories of people who have lived for years without eating. One of the most famous was Therese Neumann who died in 1963. For some thirty-five years, according to reports, the only food she consumed was Holy Communion which she received once a week. How can one explain this? Does it become possible when one reaches a high degree of sanctity or is it a miracle of God? Jack Schwarz says, 'I know such things are possible because they have been done by a number of individuals including myself ... I am eating all the time even when I am not taking in food, although not in the same way that one would normally call eating.'[15] (In his book, *Human Energy Systems* he explains how this is possible.)

For many years Schwarz has limited his food intake to three meals per week and has sometimes sustained his body for weeks with no food intake whatever. Despite the low intake – or perhaps because of it – he is a perfectly healthy man who looks far younger than he really is. Through the practice of meditation and fasting he has developed his clairvoyant and psychic abilities to a very high degree. He regards fasting as an important discipline for maintaining a high energy level necessary for healing.

The founders of the world's greatest religions, such as Jesus, Buddha, Mohammed, all recommended fasting for their followers. The gospels relate the case where the apostles returned to Jesus saying they had failed to cast out an evil spirit. Later that day, when they asked for an explanation, His response was, 'That kind of spirit is driven out only by prayer and fasting'. For many years I have wondered about this text. Now I understand fasting as an exercise which helps to make available a spiritual, or life energy, needed for healing processes.

Isolation and Meditation

In our western society we have developed a lifestyle which is overloaded with activities. Added to this, most of us live in an atmosphere in which we are constantly bombarded by stimuli, which over activate the five senses. In such an environment we run the risk of spiritual disintegration. Our psychic energies tend to become dispersed or drained. To counteract this risk we need to provide periods of isolation and confinement in our lives. Isolation from noise, from light and from people reduces the activity of the five senses and allows the sixth sense to come into operation. It provides us with an environment which enables us to recharge our spiritual energies and also facilitates the practice of meditation. Isolation and meditation have played a very important part in the development of both eastern and western spirituality.

Create Your Own Health Patterns

Over the centuries both Christian and Buddhist monks have been confining themselves to their secluded monasteries and dedicating themselves to prayer.

Healers are very much aware of the importance of confinement and meditation and today many healers spend considerable time in silent meditation before healing services. For Kathryn Kuhlman, prolonged meditation was a daily exercise. Alberto Dias, a Silva Mind Control instructor in Sao Paolo, has stated that he spends at least an hour meditating before attempting a healing. Jesus went out into the wilderness *alone* to pray. Sometimes He spent the whole night in prayer. He needed time alone to be with His Father and this was important for His own sustenance. It was also important for His own mission and was, in fact, part of His mission.

Psychics who function as mediums pass certain periods in confinement, isolated from people and events in order to enhance their mediumistic qualities. Kardec mediums in Brazil today, do not smoke, do not take alcohol, abstain from eating meat, and on days when they work, refrain from sex. Once they have been cleansed by the centre leader they even avoid shaking hands with other people.

Finally, traditional ascetic authors, various mystics and even some contemporary psychologists recommend detachment from persons and things, and especially from one's personal ego.

Chapter IV

Non-Medical Healing and Medical Science

If any of you is in trouble, he should pray; If anyone is feeling happy, he should sing a psalm. If one of you is ill, he should send for the elders of the church and they must anoint him with oil in the name of the Lord and pray over him. The prayer of faith will save the sick man and the Lord will raise him up again; and if he has committed any sins, he will be forgiven. So confess your sins to one another, and pray for one another and this will cure you.
JAMES 5: 14-16

At this point I would like to make some reflections on the relationship between natural, non-medical healing and medical science. There is no doubt twentieth century medicine has strongly coloured man's thinking on a universal level in relation to non-medical healing. In the course of the last few decades, through a gradual improvement in its techniques and a development of new and more effective types of medication, medical science has been achieving more positive and prompt results in relation to certain ailments. On the negative side, this has served to inhibit the development of man's natural healing powers, and has made him more dependent on the medical people.

Not only that, but medical science has assumed for itself a very privileged position in relation to other types of healing. The medical establishment has been opposed to unofficial types of healing and has by its very attitude cast doubt on their validity. It has outlawed certain types of healers and prescribers, and by a series of law enactments, in an effort to protect its own privileged position, it has succeeded in making some unofficial healing practices a criminal offence open to prosecution. It is no wonder that Dr Ivan Illich refers to medical science as 'the sacred cow'.[1]

Inadaquacy of Medical Science

In his book, *Nemesis Medicale*, Illich, already world-famous because of his controversial and provocative works on education, launched a devastating attack on the whole medical profession, making the bold accusation that during the last ten years medicine has killed more people than it has cured. (Nemesis is the avenging deity of the Greeks and as employed here the word means retributive justice, vengeance or chastisement.)

Illich declares that medical science, in its efforts to resolve individual ailments, amid populations gradually growing sicker, has helped to cover up the basic causes of society's illnesses, which are social, economic and cultural. It had failed to recognise that in the final analysis people are suffering from the harmful consequences of a particular life style. By helping people to bear that which is destroying them, medical science is contributing in its own way to their very destruction.

He develops his theme with some compelling arguments supported by convincing statistics drawn from the files of the medical profession itself. He claims medical science as it is today, serves little or no purpose, and has done very little for man's health during its history. Yet of all the factors which are related to man's body his life and his death, medical science is the one to which we pay most homage. It has in fact become 'the sacred cow'.

We usually attribute to medicine the increase in average lifespan, the regression of various infectious diseases and the almost total disappearance of diseases such as typhoid and tuberculosis. It is a fact that medical science perfected its treatment and made its medication more efficacious, but Illich argues that any overall improvement in health con-

Create Your Own Health Patterns

ditions was brought about essentially outside the camp of medicine. 'In almost all underdeveloped countries,' writes Charles Stewart, 'the improvement in the state of health was obtained almost totally by improving working and living conditions.[2]

Statistics show that in North American hospitals medication actually kills between sixty and one hundred and forty thousand people per year, and provokes ailments more or less grave in 3.5 million. Statistics also show that the rate of accidents in hospitals is higher than in any other industry except civil construction and mining.[3]

One of the greatest evils of medicine is that it has succeeded in making so many people dependent upon it, while it continues to deal with symptoms and to neglect the underlying causes. It destroys the autonomy of people to deal with their own health problems. An interesting statistic points to the fact that during a one-month strike in Israeli hospitals the mortality rate actually decreased, instead of increased as one would expect. Only urgent cases were admitted, which caused a general decrease of 85% in admissions. This same decrease of 85% was registered after a strike in New York hospitals, with no increase in the number of deaths.

Even early diagnosis does not seem to hold any hope. A check-up can provoke over-preoccupations with a consequent deterioration in health. Anxiety, fear or a feeling or a expectancy tends to attract that which is feared. Despite appeals for early diagnosis and periodic check-ups cancer of the breast, as a present day ailment in the United States, has assumed enormous proportions.

According to Illich, a number of studies show that these diagnostic procedures have no impact on mortality or morbidity. In fact, they tend to transform healthy people into anxious patients and he concludes that the health risks associated with this early diagnosis outweigh any actual benefits. These considerations certainly cast doubt on the whole idea of early diagnosis as a valid approach to solving health problems.

Create Your Own Health Patterns

Some Unanswered Questions

A phenomena which has become both intriguing and baffling for the medical profession is that of spontaneous remission. Without any apparent explanation so-called 'incurable diseases' heal of their own accord, contrary to medical prognosis. One of the most famous cases recorded in recent years is that of Norman Cousins, ex-editor of the *Saturday Review*, who in 1964 developed ankylosing spondylitis, a degenerative disease of the connective tissues in the spine. Cousins, who until then led a very active life and possessed a very flexible mind, was almost suddenly becoming rigid.

'The prognosis,' says Cousins, 'was progressive paralysis. I was told I'd have to make a choice between having my body freeze sitting up or lying down'. He was also told that his chance of recovery was one in five hundred. 'I didn't care,' he said, 'what the doctors said the disease was. They could have said it was cancer multiplied by ten. I would have said "OK boys, you just tend to your business; I'll tend to mine". When I discovered the disease was serious,' he tells us, 'I had a much better attitude towards it than when I thought it was transient. Before, it was something I accepted passively. I had put myself in other people's hands. Now it became a challenge. I realised I'd better get into the act and take an interest in the case.'[4]

He recalled having once read a work by Doctor Hans Seyle on how stress can adversely affect our health and actually cause sickness. Assuming that this is true, Cousins concluded that the opposite must also be true. That positive emotions like joy, happiness, excitement about living, love and hope could promote health. So he discharged himself from hospital, which he says 'is the last place someone sick should go' and booked into a hotel, taking with him lots of laughing material, films, books, magazines, plus vitamin C. He later tells us, 'I made a very interesting discovery. Ten minutes of solid belly laughter would give me two hours of painfree sleep.'[5]

It is of interest to note that some ten years later scientists discovered that the brain produces proteins called endorphins, which are natural painkillers, and their production is triggered by laughter and a general state of excitement.[6]

Cousins discovered that because of the anaesthetic effect of laughter he was able to dispense with not only the painkillers, but also the sleeping pills and this allowed the natural healing powers of the body to function without interference.

He tells us 'At the end of the critical two weeks, during which I took the love, laughter and ascorbic-acid (vitamin C) therapy, I was able to move my thumbs and I knew I was going to make it all the way.'[7]

Traditional medicine has difficulty in explaining the Cousins case. Some doctors would say 'Yes, he was that one in five hundred chance'. But what was it that made him the one in five hundred? There have been thousands of cases of spontaneous remission over the years, but what is fascinating about the Cousins case is that it did not just happen. After hearing the doctors fatalistic prognosis he consciously decided to take himself in hand and did what he thought best to bring about his recovery. The remission of the illness was spontaneous once he provided the conditions necessary for recovery.

This type of phenomena and many others continue to question medical science, challenging its concepts and its methods. About two hundred cases of remission of terminal cancer have actually been published. Prayer groups claim to have replaced lost teeth and restored withered limbs.

How does one explain the many cases of heart attack upon losing one's job? The number of cases of serious illness following divorce?

Why did the ex-Shah of Iran, Reza Pahlavi and ex-President of the United States, Richard Nixon, both contract serious illnesses at a time of personal political crisis?

How does one explain the case of the Irish girl who

pines away after her lover has left for a foreign land and the Biafran who dies within hours of becoming aware that a voodoo curse has been put on him?

Why does one cigarette smoker get cancer and another equally heavy smoker does not? Why is it that in a community where all eat basically the same food, breathe the same air and share the same lifestyle, don't all get cancer? Flu is caused by virus, why is it that some are infected by it while others in the same household are not?

These are some of the questions that official science has not adequately answered or has tended to ignore.

The Future of Medicine

At this stage we may ask the question: will medical science ever reach a stage of development where it will control all illness? This may still be a dream of some medical people, but a dream which, I believe, will never become a reality for two reasons. First, while medical science continues to operate within its own narrow confines, treating physical symptoms of a deeper sickness, it will never solve society's illnesses. Secondly, as long as man has a need to be ill and his illness serves a purpose for him, then he will defy the most brilliant medical practitioner.

Through the history of medical science we note that there has always been some disease or group of diseases outside of its reach.

During the last one hundred years dramatic changes have occurred in the nature of disease afflicting western society. First, industrialisation sparked epidemics of infectious diseases which subsided at a certain point in time. Then tuberculosis took over for a period and, in turn, declined, before either its cause had been discovered or treatment programmes had been initiated. This in turn was replaced by major malnutrition syndromes – rickets and pellagra – which peaked and declined to be replaced by early childhood diseases which in turn gave way to duodenal ulcers. Now modern epidemics take their toll – coronary disease, hypertension, cancer, arthritis, diabetes and mental disorders.

It seems as if, deprived of our old diseases, we have invented new ones which seem to manifest some essential disfunction at the very core of our being.

John Cassels, Professor of Epidermology at the University of North Carolina, points out that the decline of these ailments seemed to happen independently of the medical field. The conclusion he draws is that diseases appear and disappear in relation to factors such as food, housing conditions, physical and mental hygiene and working conditions.[8]

Today there seems to be a tremendous increase in stress-related diseases, a fact which may be explained in part by a change in our understanding of disease. Many illnesses which formerly were not regarded as psychosomatic are now being understood as having at least some emotional components.

Doctor Ken Pelletier, professor at the School of Medicine at the University of California says, 'If you look at the most recent literature in the field you may even conclude that virtually all states of health are to some degree psychosomatic. The four major categories of disease in the United States today – cardiovascular disease, cancer, arthritis and respiratory disorders – are increasingly seen as psychosomatic. I think that virtually all viral infections are stress-related, virtually all inflammatory disorders are stress-related. The only disorders that are not are traumatic injuries – accidents.'[9] On second thoughts he admits that even accidents could be due to stress. For example, a husband may break his leg at the time of a divorce as a way of communicating to his wife that he really needs her. Of course, he does not choose this way consciously or deliberately. But he is in conflict, looking for a way out, searching for a solution and the answer comes. He unconsciously may have provoked the accident and though it is not the type of solution he wants, it may be the 'blessing in disguise'.

Disease, according to Dupuy and Karsenty[10] is a type of 'strike', a passive protest of the body against a situation that has become intolerable. The digestive problems, the headaches, the rheumatic pains and the depressive states are above all else healthy protests of an ill-treated organism. They are an expression of man's inability to cope with his living situation or with himself. Modern man has a need to be ill. He cannot cope, so illness serves a purpose for him.

A few years ago in Brazil, Dr Christian Barnard was able to fill one of the major football stadiums twice on the same day with crowds who hysterically acclaimed his ability to exchange human hearts. Did he really effect anything for the health of the patient? I feel that if an individual succeeds in destroying his own heart, kidney or other vital organ for some reason unknown to medical science, then the chances are that, given enough time, he will also destroy or reject the substitute heart or kidney.

The Relationship of Environment to Health

When I speak of disease as a manifestation of an internal conflict I am very much aware that many of our conflicts are related to our environment. For this reason when I conceive the possibility of living a life free of sickness, I am presuming the existence of a normal healthy environment. The human person needs to eat sufficient healthful food, breathe clean air and take sufficient rest. But unfortunately our environment is often more disease provoking than health giving.

Poor physical environment must be considered one of the greatest hazards to health. Polluted air, contaminated water, unhealthful diet, improper sanitation are all acknowledged as causes of a very high percent of disease. Since this is so, the general health problems will not be solved in the hospitals or in the pharmacies. Health authorities must face

Create Your Own Health Patterns

the fundamental problem and be prepared to put much more emphasis and resources to work at the environmental level.

Recently I met a realistic young nurse who went through a variety of nursing experiences both in hospitals and in public health. At a certain point in her career she decided to quit working in such structures and instead involve herself directly with the people in a poor area in the periphery of Sao Paolo. When I asked her what led to the decision she spoke of the frustration of working in a situation such as hospital where one is so much out of touch with the environmental factor, to which so many illnesses are directly linked. She mentioned the all-too-common occurrence of the child who is admitted to the hospital suffering from anaemia, is effectively treated and within a week is re-admitted suffering from the same illness. There is a vicious circle involved here. Anaemia is the result of worms caused by improper sanitation due to a lack of money and education.

This young lady took the logical step of going to the source of the problem. It is encouraging to know that many of the young doctors graduating from medical school today are applying themselves to the problem in the same way. It remains a challenge to be faced realistically, by idealistic people, who are willing to confront one of the most urgent social problems of our time.

Under the concept of environment I include the political and economic environment. Man has a basic human instinct for self-preservation and when this is threatened, as may occur in the case of severe economic crisis or war, then sickness can follow. Man also has a basic human instinct for self-determination and self-expression. When this need is frustrated, as for example, in an environment where there is prolonged political repression or lack of freedom of expression, then illness, both mental and physical, can ensue.

It is generally agreed that persons who enjoy more internal harmony, those who are more 'at ease with themselves', are less prone to 'disease' and have a better chance of

Create Your Own Health Patterns

surviving, even in an unfavourable environment. On the other hand, illness can occur in a healthy environment if the person is in conflict within himself. A person needs to live in complete harmony not only with one's self but also with one's total environment, with other people, with social structures and with nature itself. Humans need to live in a community of love, where there is an environment of peace, harmony and security and where each member is recognised, accepted and appreciated.

When relationships are not harmonious, sickness – both mental or physical – may result. Hatred, resentment, bad relationships cause sickness and this sickness is liable to persist until the underlying causes are corrected.

For this reason the healing of relationships and the replacement of negative feelings by love has become a very important process in my healing services. Psychologists know well that when a husband or wife comes to the clinic with an ailment related to a tense relationship, the problem will not be solved until the underlying cause, the ailing relationship, is healed. When parents bring a disturbed child for help the experienced family counsellor knows that the disturbance is merely a symptom of a deeper problem of relationship, and can be cured only by healing within the context of the whole family. The baby who cries constantly may not be hungry or physically uncomfortable but simply responding to a tense relationship between its father and mother.

Frank points out that, in general, western industrialised society sees illness as the malfunctioning of the body, to be corrected by the appropriate medical intervention. Some believe that the cause of mental illness lies in some form of derangements of the brain. If these things are so, the physician becomes a highly skilled scientist-technician whose job it is to diagnose the illness and correct it, much as the auto mechanic deals with a broken-down car.[11]

Writing on this topic, Frank states, 'While this approach to illness has scored notable successes and undoubtedly will score many more, it is seriously deficient in a crucial respect. It fails to acknowledge that psychological and bodily processes can profoundly affect each other. High among the former are illnesses emerging from the interplay of the sick person with his family and his culture.'[12] He goes on to show that while emotional problems can cause various physiological ailments, so also can bodily ailments give rise to a variety of problems – emotional, familiar, cultural and moral – affecting the individual. The sick person, for example, becomes separated from his social environment and from his friends. Prolonged illness often causes depression. Constant misery gives rise to anxiety, frustration and finally despair, and all this affects one's self esteem.

With Collaboration a New Hope is Born

While I accept Illich's central themes as being valid, and find his well-documented evidence convincing, still I cannot agree with his overall attitude, which is in effect, a total condemnation of the official medical world. Medical science may be responsible for killing many people, making many others ill, ignoring the underlying causes of illness, and conditioning people's thinking to the point of making whole societies dependent upon it. Nevertheless, it must be admitted that medical science has helped keep many people alive who would otherwise have died, and has been instrumental in restoring many people to health.

I see an urgent need for co-operation between the different categories involved in healing – the medical healers, the psychological healers and the unofficial healers. Man is not a body, he is not a mind, he is not a spirit. He exists on three levels all at once – physical, mental and spiritual. Medicine concerns itself directly with the physical part of man but the causes of most of man's illness are of a nonphysical nature. Psychologists in general, work with the mind, while unofficial healers tend to work through the spiritual part of man. With more understanding of the others' field and added co-operation between the different healing systems, many benefits would accrue.

The non-medical healers, who actually minister to more clients than do the medical people, tend to see illness more as a disorder of the whole person, involving not only his body but his mind, his emotions and his relationship with others. For them, the intense personal relationship with the patient becomes an important factor in the healing process.

Because of its own shortcomings medical science has actually contributed to the building up of a flourishing community of unorthodox healers. The insensitivity of medical science to the more fundamental causes – emotional and environmental – of many ailments, and the effects of these ailments on the patient, 'account for many of its failures, and impels the ill to seek out forms of healing which operate on a different premise.'[13] Dr B. Inglis, author of *The Case for Unorthodox Medicine*, states that people do not visit a fringe practitioner because they are gullible, stupid or superstitious, though they may be; they go to him because they think or hope that they can get something from him that their doctor no longer gives. They are right; often the doctor does not pretend to be able to give it.[14]

Illich proposes the deprofessionalisation of medicine. 'This does not imply negation of specialised healers, of competence, of mutual criticism or of public control. It does imply a bias against mystification, against transnational dominance of one orthodox view, against disbarment of healers chosen by their patients but not certified by the guild.'[15]

It is encouraging to note the increasing co-operation, especially among the younger generation, between the medical, psychological and unofficial healers. Many doctors recommend mental therapy or counselling for their clients, and I recently heard of some cases where doctors even prescribe psychic or spiritual healing. The Sunday *San Francisco Chronicle* of 22 July, 1975, carried an article on a Bay Area doctor, Jerry Bronstein, who is an emergency room physician at Kaiser Hospital in Hayward and also is a spiritual healer with the Gentle Brothers and Sisters, a healing group in Berkeley.[16]

At the University of California Medical Centre, San Francisco, some doctors are encouraging patients suffering from ailments, such as cancer and arthritis, to meditate on the affected area of the body and to send it healing power. According to their observations the results are positive.

Krippner and Villoldo cite the case of Toshio Yamamoto, a medical doctor who is director of an 800 bed hospital in Japan. He has a group of eighty healers whose services are available to the patients, and he himself has claimed that quite a number of patients for whom medical science has no answer have subsequently responded to the healers approach and have been cured.[17]

An interesting and significant development recently took place in England. The British National Federation of Spiritual Healers obtained permission from the Minister for Health to allow its members to visit patients in some 1,500 hospitals throughout the country. Upon request from a patient, the hospital authorities get in touch with the Federation and ask for the presence of a healer.[18]

Traditionally priest and ministers in most countries have been free to visit hospitals with or without the patient's request and give 'spiritual assistance'. In fact, many hospitals have their own official chaplains. What is significant in this new development is the official recognition of the presence of a person on the medical platform, in the capacity of a 'healer' as opposed to a 'minister'. Only a short time ago the World Federation of Healing set up its headquarters in London University and one of its aims is to make healers available to hospital patients worldwide.[19]

Another interesting development is the use of paradiagnostics in the medical field. Earlier I mentioned the use of psychics or mediums for diagnostic purposes in non-medical healing. 'The "paradiagnostic" differs from the medium in that he diagnoses at a distance, through clairvoyance, without any contact with the patient. This is being used by a number of doctors throughout the world, including the Soviet Union and the United States, but as yet is very much on the experimental level.'[20]

One such experiment was carried out by Dr Norman Shealy, director of the Pain Rehabilitation Clinic in La Crosse, Wisconsin. Using psychic Henry Rucker for diagnostic purposes, Shealy claims he was 80% accurate in tests involving 350 patients.[21] Another such experiment was carried out by a doctor at the University of Tennessee College of Medicine. He also claims an 80% degree of accuracy, according to Shealy.[22]

Some psychotherapists and psychologists today suspect that cancer may be caused at least in part by psychological factors. Dr E. P. Pendergrass, a past president of the American Cancer Society, has stated that 'there is solid evidence that the course of cancer is often affected by emotional distress.'[23] Doctors are having recourse more and more to psychological procedures in their battle to conquer cancer.

A very interesting study was done by Dr O. C. Simonton, a radiologist at the Cancer Counselling and Research Centre Fort Worth, Texas, who has done pioneering research in this field. In the course of his work with cancer patients his curiosity was aroused by two recurring factors. One was the many cases of spontaneous remission – recovery from the disease with no apparent explanation – and two, the many cases where patients would make correct predictions about the outcome of an illness, which at times ran contrary to all medical prognosis. For example, 'I will not die until I see my son safely home from the war in Vietnam.'[24] He concluded that there must be some psychological factors at work.

Another factor that intrigued Simonton was that he would give two patients, with the same diagnosis and similar backgrounds, the same treatment and get widely divergent results. 'Here I was,' he says, 'in a position of being responsible for telling people how they would respond to treatment and I knew that I couldn't predict. So I started to ask

Create Your Own Health Patterns

them why they thought they responded in the way they did. What I heard from them had to do with attitudes, goals in life and some relatively intangible things that lumped together made a lot of folksy nonsense. I was able to piece together what I learned,' Simonton says, 'and develop something that could help patients help themselves improve their chances of getting well. Overcoming medically incurable cancer,' he remarks, 'is a very difficult task. It's doing the impossible.'[25] Nevertheless he has been getting results about twice as good as those obtained by conventional treatment. His approach represents a radical departure from the traditional medical mode. Asking the patients such questions as 'What do you think is causing that?' and 'Why do you think you are responding as you are?' and taking their answers seriously, is certainly unconventional.

In his treatment of cancer Simonton has developed a process (which is familiar to graduates of Silva Mind Control) in which the patients are taught to visualise the cancer cells or tumours, picturing them in their 'mind's eye' or on a 'mental screen'. They are directed, for example, to visualise an army of white blood cells swarming over the cancer, carrying off the malignant cells that had been weakened or destroyed by the radiation treatment if radiation treatment had been used. Each patient uses his own creative imagination to work on the process. One woman, for example, saw the white blood cells as a vacuum cleaner sucking the cancerous cells away. A young boy visualised cowboys using lassos made of white blood cells capturing the cancer cells which were seen as the bandits, and destroying them. A big part of Simonton's work now consists of training his patients in the use of this visualisation process.[26]

Lawrence Le Shan, a psychologist, trained psychic and healer in the United States, has found in his research, that most cancer patients suffer an emotional trauma six to eighteen months prior to the onset of the ailment. Working on Le Shan's findings, Simonton regresses his patients to that event, puts them in touch with it, and helps them to re-orient their lives from there. In studying 152 cases over a two-year period he noted that response to treatment was directly related to two factors: having a positive attitude and practising the visualisation faithfully.[27]

In accepting the 1973 Nobel Prize for Physiology and Medicine, Nikolas Tinbergen states, 'The more that is being discovered about psychosomatic diseases, and in general, about the extremely complex two-way traffic between the brain and the rest of the body, the more obvious it has become that a too rigid distinction between mind and body is only of limited use to medical science.' Tinbergen concludes that if this division is maintained by medicine 'it can be a hindrance to its advance'.[28]

As I was writing these pages I got a phone call from a friend, Arlis, telling me the good news about Barbara. 'She is home and well.' Barbara, a young woman of twenty-four, developed a uterine infection. Later it transferred to an ovary in the form of a cyst. She did not respond to antibiotics taken orally so she was put on I V treatment. Her condition gradually deteriorated to the point of being threatened with septicemia and she ended up in intensive care for two days. At this stage the doctors decided on a hysterectomy as a last resort and scheduled the operation for Thursday morning. This was a big decision for Barbara since her whole future as a potential mother was at question. On Monday evening, a friend of hers brought in a scientologist who worked on her for a short time. On Tuesday the doctors noted a marked improvement and on Wednesday they decided to cancel the operation, and began to speak of the phenomenal recovery in terms of a miracle. The interesting factor is that all the scientologist attempted to do was help the girl to relax and remove certain blockages so that medication prescribed by the doctors could do what it was intended to do. This for me is one example of how much the healing professions need each other and how much they can achieve through co-operation.

In Sao Paolo I became acquainted with the parapsychology clinic Mens Sana, directed by Frei Albino Garibaldi, where sensitives are used for diagnostic purposes with clients suffering from both mental and physical ailments. The sensitives are usually females who have a high degree of psychic ability and they play a role somewhat similar to the medium in the spiritist centre. The usual procedure is that the sensitive sits close to the client, gets into a relaxed or mild hypnotic state, and then, under the direction of the parapsychologist, describes what she is picking up from the client. Then, using the information received, the parapsychologist proceeds with his treatment. Sometimes the sensitive orientates the parapsychologist in the treatment process. It is interesting to note that these sensitives achieve a high degree of accuracy in what they pick up.

There are other experiments of the same nature being carried out in Brazilian clinics run by doctors, psychiatrists and parapsychologists. At the Institute Brasileiro de Parasicologia Clinica, Dr Eliezer C. Mendes uses sensitives for both diagnosis and treatment of emotional and physical disturbances. Both the client and the sensitive get into a hypnotic state, and the disturbed personality of the patient is taken on by the sensitive. The actual scene which led to the disturbance is usually acted out, and during the process the client is healed of the disturbance. A complete cure can take anything from one to thirty sessions. Dr Mendes understands the disturbance as sometimes due to a trauma suffered at an earlier stage in life, and sometimes due to a trauma inherited from a past life.

Harold Sherman[29] quotes a very interesting case where he elicited the co-operation of a doctor to effect a spiritual healing. When he was a young man back in the twenties he developed a gangrene in one of his toes. It reached the point of endangering his life, and he was scheduled for amputation of his leg. This he did not want. On the evening prior to the operation he attempted to bring about a healing by using the visualisation technique of seeing his toe in a normal, healthy condition. But the pain was so excruciating that he found himself totally incapable of visualising his toe well. During the doctor's evening visit Sherman explained to him what he was attempting to do and how he was failing completely because of a lack of faith. He asked the doctor to help with the request, 'When you get home tonight, will you sit quietly by yourself for half an hour and picture in your mind what has to happen to my toe to make it well?' The doctor, who was his close friend, promised that he would and so the time was set. At the appointed time, Sherman simply tried to relax himself as much as possible while the doctor did the visualisation for him, and to the surprise of everybody the miracle happened. By morning the infection in the toe had burst open, drained itself, and the toe was healed.

This was certainly a most unusual way of gaining the co-operation of the doctor to achieve a spiritual healing. Some psychic schools of healing believe that doctors, nurses and others involved in the healing profession possess special healing powers. They would even go so far as to say that the mere presence of the doctors has a healing effect on the patient. (This actually has been the experience of many people.) They seem to think that it occurs through the intermingling of the energy bodies, or auras, when the doctor and patient come within a certain degree of proximity to each other.

Francis MacNutt speaks of a prayer group in St Louis, where several doctors pray for their patients before, during and after operations, and states, 'The beautiful thing is that they, too, have seen cures wrought through prayer when they came to the limits of their medical art. At other times, doctors, relatives, and friends have visited hospitals to pray for their patients. Some underwent successful operations; others were not even operated on, for the growth disappeared, or the condition was cleared up beforehand.'[30]

Speaking of the relation between non-medical healing and medicine, Ambrose and Olga Worrall state, 'We never interfere with medical treatment. We insist that physicians be consulted in all cases. We believe prayer and medicine do not stand unalterably opposed. We can work with doctors; we are not against them. Spiritual healing, like all healing, is only a technique for achieving wholeness, and all wholeness is of God.

'We recognise that in practically every case of illness, medical or other treatment has been administered before spiritual healing is tried; that in cases where recovery follows both spiritual healing and medical treatment, it may be the result of the two methods. Therefore, we do not give all the credit to spiritual healing. We believe spiritual healers should work in association with other healing professions.

'We would also like to make clear that healing has not and does not occur in every case of spiritual therapy. Why it occurs is a mystery. The only answer to this, quite frankly and bluntly, is that we do not know. Neither do the physicians in many cases.'[31]

In the old testament the Book of Ecclesiasticus (Sirach) has some words of wisdom to say about healing:

Hold the physician in honour, for he is essential to you,
    and God it was who established his profession.
From God the doctor has his wisdom,
    and the king provides for his sustenance.
His knowledge makes the doctor distinguished,
    and gives him access to those in authority.
God makes the earth yield healing herbs
    which the prudent man should not neglect;
Was not the water sweetened by a twig
    that men might learn his power?
He endows men with the knowledge
    to glory in his mighty works,
Through which the doctor eases pain
    and the druggist prepares his medicines;
Thus God's creative work continues without cease
    in its efficacy on the surface of the earth.
My son, when you are ill, delay not,
    but pray to God, who will heal you:

Create Your Own Health Patterns

> Flee wickedness; let your hands be just,
>   cleanse your heart of every sin;
> Offer your sweet-smelling oblation and petition,
>   a rich offering according to your means.
> Then give the doctor his place
>   lest he leave; for you need him too.
> There are times that give him an advantage,
>   and he too beseeches God
> That his diagnosis may be correct
>   and his treatment bring about a cure.
> He who is a sinner toward his Maker
>   will be defiant toward the doctor.
>   (Sir. 38: 1-15).[32]

Here we have a recommendation to pray to God for healing in time of sickness. The role of the doctor, the druggist and the use of herbs are emphasised, and finally the need for inner healing, because the person in conflict or disharmony may defy the healer.

CHAPTER V

Inner Healing

*Do all you can to preserve the unity of the
Spirit by the peace that binds you together*
EPHESIANS 4:3

Some people wonder if sickness is the result of sin or if there is some connection between the two. Sin is often described as a transgression against the law of God. The law of God is the law of nature; what theologians call the 'Natural Law'. It is a law inherent in God's creation, a law of total harmony; harmony between people and God, between human beings and between humans and the animal, plant and inanimate kingdoms. When we act contrary to these laws or interfere with them in any way, we suffer the consequences both in the moral and the physical order. The moral consequence is what we call sin and the physical consequence is disease. It is not that God chastises us for our wrongdoing but rather that when we act against nature we suffer the consequences of our own actions. Nature, as it were, hits back at us. This does not necessarily mean that sick people are guilty of sin or are morally responsible for what is happening to them.

MacNutt speaks of the connection between sickness and sin, stating in effect, that physical sickness is a sign that we are not OK with our neighbour. 'The connection of sin and sickness,' he says, 'is now being brought to our attention again, remarkably not by the church, but by psychologists and doctors who recognise that much, if not most, physical sickness has an emotional component.'[1]

Assuming that illness, in general, comes from somewhere inside of the person, from wrong thinking, emotional conflict or lack of harmonious integration with one's group, then it follows that for complete and permanent healing, inner healing is necessary. The manifestation of the illness, whether it be organic or functional, is the symptom. The underlying cause often remains safely hidden. When we treat only the symptoms, leaving the cause of the ailment untouched, the chances are that the symptoms may reappear or merely become transferred.

A major criticism of behaviourist therapy is that it works with symptoms and may or may not touch the cause. It is basically a conditioning process, and in psychological jargon is referred to as behaviour modification. Surprisingly those who work with this type of therapy claim they get very good results. They also claim that through symptom treatment, the underlying cause, in many cases, disappears or is affected in some mysterious way.

Whether the medical profession is prescribing mediation or performing an operation, it is still working on the external manifestation of an inner sickness. That is why we so often witness a recurrence of an ailment, even after seemingly successful surgery. In many instances operations and medications effect complete and permanent healings. Could it be, that through working on the symptom, the underlying cause is also affected? Perhaps through the incision of the knife and all the accompanying pain and stress, the patient is induced to let go of that which is the source of the ailment? Perhaps this is the opportunity to take time out and put things together in his or her life, to establish inner peace and harmony and to become reconciled with others.

It is recognised that the doctor who takes time to talk to his or her patients, to learn about their background or what may be going on inside them, gets better results.

Dr Takashi Enokibara, a physician from Dracena in the state of Sao Paolo, Brazil, likes to describe himself as a 'family doctor'. His particular interest is responding to the health needs of the whole family. This experience with families has led him to the conclusion that many health problems are related to conflict and strife within the home. Sickness is more frequent in homes where there is a lack of understanding, little sensitivity, poor acceptance, and where the flow of love is cut off. Not being a family counsellor, Dr Takashi felt frustrated. His inability to deal with the core problem led him to the concept of a therapeutic community, which he visualises as a type of clinic or healing centre where a doctor, a psychologist (or counsellor) and a spiritual healer (or advisor) would work together, in an effort to effect both external and internal healing in the clients.

Looking back on my ministry I realise that for many years I attempted to heal people on a very superficial level. A case in question is the use of the sacrament of Penance. People came to confession, recited their sins, expressed their sorrow, and I gave them absolution. The process sometimes appeared to me as a weekly or monthly house-cleaning. The need to repeat the cleaning operation continued week after week, month after month, but fundamentally nothing seemed to change in the penitent's lifestyle. Because of the confessional environment, together with my own inability to understand the depth of some of the problems, I very often applied the orientation I got in the seminary, encouraging the penitent to try again, to use will power, and to count on the grace of God. Unfortunately, in many cases this did not work, and for me this ministry often became a very frustrating activity.

Once again, I was dealing with symptoms and there was no inner healing. I was not getting to the root of the problem, and consequently there was no significant change in the penitent's life. What help could I give to the teenage girl suffering from chronic depression, stemming from a very poor self image, who had just attempted suicide for the third time? How could I help the scrupulous penitent, who because of a feeling of guilt, returned to confess the same sins week after week. These people were suffering great pain and I was not able to help them in an effective way.

I was fully aware, at the time, that preaching repentance was not enough. It often served to make people feel guiltier. Yes, I was able to give them my time, my understanding and my concern, and these were often a help. I was also able to refer some cases for professional help, but that was as far as I was able to go.

On the positive side, the frustration of dealing with such cases, together with my own sense of inadequacy lured me back to study again. I realise now that many of the foregoing problems are involuntary, and although often deeply embedded in the subconscious mind, they can, nevertheless, be solved.

When is inner healing necessary? I believe that we all need inner healing continuously, especially emotional and spiritual healings. This can happen in various ways. Being among people who are accepting, understanding and empathetic has a healing effect. Praying, alone or with others, is often a powerful healing experience. Being aware of others, extending a helping hand, saying a kind word, or writing a loving letter are all healing processes. In fact, most of us are constantly healing and being healed by others.

But, there are certain times in life when inner healing becomes a matter of urgency. At times our very survival demands it. According to MacNutt, 'Inner healing is indicated when we become aware that we are held down in any way by hurts of the past. We all suffer from this kind of bondage to one degree or another. Some severely, some minimally.'[2] Some people, for example, suffer from a sense of failure in life, which gives birth to a hopelessness about the future. Others suffer from deep anxiety, unfounded fears, or deep depression.

Psychologists tell us that most of the hurts stem from the forgotten past – the early years of childhood. In some cases the hurt can be traced to the prenatal stage. The experience of some healing groups seem to corroborate this opinion. MacNutt states, 'There is a good deal of evidence that some hurt goes back even before birth while the child was still being carried in the mother's womb ... If the mother does not really want the child or is suffering from anxiety or fear, the infant seems somehow to pick up the feelings of the mother and to respond to them ... The earliest memories up to the time we are two or three years old seem to be the most important in setting patterns for our future behaviour.'[3] In these situations there is need for inner healing.

Inner healing, in general, is the healing of the 'inner man'. By the 'inner man' I mean the intellectual, volitional and affective make-up of every person. It involves getting in touch with self, changing one's attitudes and healing past memories and emotional hurts.

The idea of living in harmony is confusing for some people. They don't know what it means nor how to achieve it. Being in harmony does not mean trying to please everybody, nor accepting situations with which one does not agree. Neither does it mean presenting a semblance of peace, wearing a mask or a plastic smile. It does imply being totally honest with self and the other. It implies having one's own particular viewpoint and being able to communicate it. It also implies being in touch with one's own inner feelings and possessing the ability and courage to express them openly and honestly.

Anger, for example, is a problem for many people. Being angry is seen by some as sinful. Parents try to teach their children not to be angry although they think it is all right for them to be angry. 'Nice people don't get angry', they say. People attempt to hide it, but they never succeed, because anger manifests itself despite their most determined efforts at concealing it. It manifests itself in one's behaviour and through one's body language. It betrays itself in the facial expression and in the very tone of voice used to conceal it. If there is any sin in anger it is in the dishonesty of not communicating it. Anger means conflict, tension and frustration, but in the expression of the anger resides the resolution of the conflict. Concealed anger kills the spirit and simultaneously kills the body.

Create Your Own Health Patterns

Healing of Memories

Memory plays a very central role in our lives. Today's perceptions are all coloured by our memories of the past. Our present patterns of behaviour are determined to a great extent by our memories of the past. Our reactions to situations and people, our feelings of joy and sorrow, grief and anxiety are all linked to our memories. The memories of the past seem to be more important than the actual events of the past. What remains with us today is not the event, but the memory of it and the feeling which that memory evokes. In short, what remains today is our experience of the past event. Different people experience the same event in different ways. Different people have different memories and feelings about the same event. Most of our emotional reactions are closely linked with our memories.

People in the healing professions all realise how important memories are, which explains why they ask questions such as, 'What's been going on in your life? What's been happening to you? Where did that come from?'

Much of our suffering is tied in with painful memories. We hurt and we need healing. Feelings of separation, loneliness, alienation, anxiety and fear are the results of painful memories.

It is interesting to note what we do with memories. We like to carry the pleasant memories with us, while we prefer to bury the painful ones. Our normal response to undesirable memories is to forget them. 'Let's forget it'. 'Let's not talk about it anymore'. In fact some of our past memories are so painful, that we succeed in blocking them out completely from our conscious mind. But alas, blocking them out does not mean that we are rid of them. We simply repress them into the subconscious mind and they remain with us as part of the 'baggage' we carry through life.

Psychologists tell us that it is really the subconscious that is in command in our lives. Most of our behaviour is automatic. We tend to react instead of acting. We are victims of situations instead of being in charge of our own affairs. We need to change from automatic pilot to manual control.

Repressed or forgotten memories become an independent vital force in our lives and exert a crippling effect on our behaviour. While they remain forgotten they are no longer available to the conscious mind and our ability to change and grow is impeded. The reason we repeat so many failures of the past, whether as an individual, a class, or a nation is due to forgotten memories. We tend to lose touch with the past – our most learned teacher – and so we block our growth.

Among the spiritual healers, Agnes Stanford is one of the greatest proponents of what she terms 'Healing of the Memories'.[4] This entails bringing to light the buried, unpleasant, memories of the past and healing the emotional scars caused by the traumatic experiences associated with those memories.

According to MacNutt the idea is to call up or call to light those hidden memories and 'heal them from the wounds that still remain and affect their present lives, draining the poison of past hurts and resentment, and filling with love all those places in them that have been empty for so long.'[5]

In his book, *Inner healing*, Michael Scanlon speaks of the importance of healing what he calls 'root memories', noting, for example, that 'a childhood memory of being alone at night in the dark, being lost amidst the crowd or being unwanted by parents, could be the foundation for a later fear of darkness, of strangers or of intimacy. Memories of a tyrannical father can be the root of many subsequent bad authority experiences'.[6] If only the actual manifestations of the deeper problem are dealt with then there is a real need for inner healing.

How do we heal those wounded memories? The first step is to get in touch with them and make them available. They are part of us and part of our life's history. Getting in touch with them is already part of the healing. This may be achieved through prayer, reflection, or meditation, but more often it happens through the assistance of a third party ... psychologist, counsellor, prayer group or even one's own family.

I remember speaking to a lady – the youngest of a family of five – who for many years had been suffering from a very deep feeling of rejection. On occasions she felt she didn't even have a right to exist. She had built up an acute sensitivity in this area and was constantly constructing situations to test her degree of acceptance by others. One situation after another confirmed that she was the unwanted one and served only to intensify her feeling of rejection. She suspected she was an unwanted child and had a particularly strong antipathy towards her mother. The sense of rejection often led to fits of deep depression with suicidal tendencies. Having wrestled with the problem for a long time she finally decided to put the question to her mother. 'What were the circumstances surrounding my birth?' Her mother confirmed her suspicion, explaining that her conception was in fact an accident and was not 'meant to be'. Economically they could not afford to have any more children at the time and it would have meant moving to a larger house. She also spoke of the suffering she went through – the frustration, the conflict and the anxiety.

The conversation was beneficial to both mother and daughter. The daughter became more accepting of herself, became more in control of what was going on inside of her, and her relationship with her mother improved remarkably.

Forgiveness and Resentment

Earlier I quoted the case of the 'miraculous' cure of Jack Schwarz at the moment he made a total act of forgiveness (cf. Chap I). This suggests that letting go of negative feelings has a healing effect on the person. At that moment harmony is re-established. One becomes re-aligned with God's harmonious creation. One becomes at-one.

Create Your Own Health Patterns

MacNutt quotes the testimony of two people after a communal penance service, in which the emphasis was on forgiveness of enemies. 'One was a man who had suffered constant chest pain, since undergoing open heart surgery. During the communal penance when he was asked to think of someone who had hurt him, he thought of his boss, a man he regarded as unjust. At first he wasn't going to forgive him, but then with all the time allowed, he entered into a prayer of forgiveness. At that moment all the painful effects of the open heart surgery left him.'[7] The other was a case of a young woman whose pylonidal cyst disappeared instantly the moment she was able to repent of a deep-seated grudge.

In the Lord's Prayer we ask the Father to 'forgive us our offences as we forgive those who offend us'. Forgiving is healing. To the degree that we forgive, we heal. We restore harmony. We heal ourselves and others because they too are touched by our forgiveness. In His preaching Jesus emphasised the need to forgive. 'You have learned how it was said; "An eye for an eye and a tooth for a tooth!" But I say this to you; offer the wicked man no resistance. On the contrary, if anyone hits you on the right cheek offer him the other as well' (Mt. 5: 38-39).

His final expression of forgiveness, when He asked His Father to forgive His torturers, was very significant. 'Father, forgive them, for they know not what they do.' At that moment He was in total harmony with self and everyone. It was His final 'letting go of'. He had already let go of everything in this world, and this final act left Him free to resurrect, since nothing on this earth held Him bound anymore.

Today it is generally agreed that negative feelings, when harboured over a period of time, have a detrimental effect on our mental and physical health. Feelings of anxiety and fear affect the stomach area and can produce ulcers. Of course this is nothing new. But what *is* new is the suggestion that many heart problems are related to a love that is misdirected or cut off. A love that has ceased to flow is capable of destroying the very organ which is its life source. Also new is the suggestion of certain researchers that cancer is related to negative feelings, especially resentment and anger.

In their book, *Psychosomatics: How Your Emotions Can Damage Your Health*, Howard and Martha Lewis state: 'Even cancer has recently been linked to emotion. Researchers are finding that cancer victims are often people who have long felt hopeless and have believed that their lives are doomed to despair. The onset of the disease in many cases is associated with a series of overwhelming losses that make a person finally give up entirely.'[8]

Speaking of the connection between negative feelings and colitis they state: 'Ulcerative colitis is thought to develop when a predisposed person fails to express chronic resentment and anger. On an unconscious level the mucous membrane of his colon responds to these repressed emotions. The ensuing engorgement and hyperactivity produces bleeding ... Ulcerative colitis is often accompanied by severe depression and a feeling of hopelessness and despair. The typical victim is immature and dependent, particularly on his mother. He often is perfectionistic and rigid and tends to be wary of other people.'[9]

Healing of Relationships

Inner healing of relationships has become an important part of my healing services. The people involved are directed to become aware, in so far as they can, of any bad or negative feelings. This is effected through a fantasy trip, using visualisation and the help of a guide. The guide can be anyone who serves as a model or a type of consultant for the individual concerned. For many people the guide is Jesus Christ. In the course of the trip all the people with whom relations have broken down are visited mentally. Peace and harmony are restored. It is not sufficient to let go of bad feelings. One has to replace them with love. Love needs to communicate itself. It has to be allowed to flow and touch everybody and everything.

Create Your Own Health Patterns

Signs of Inner Healing

According to spiritual healers, inner healing is sometimes experienced in a very dramatic manner. It very often brings about a significant change in the person's life. It may lead to more acceptance of self and of others. Sometimes one achieves more openness, deeper trust and renewed courage. There is often a new sense of freedom, an added excitement about living. One begins to live less in the past and future and more in the present. There is often a greater sense of feeling loved, together with a deeper desire to love others. There is usually a deeper sense of peace, harmony and tranquility which become permanent realities in one's life.

Writing of this peace and harmony, Erich Fromm makes reference to the Messianic view of peace which he describes as a state of 'harmony between man and man, man and woman, and man and nature ... It can be obtained only if man develops fully in order to become truly human, if he is capable of loving, if he knows truth and does justice, if he develops his power of reasoning to the point which frees him from the bondage of man and from the bondage of irrational passions ... It is the accomplishment of true harmony and union; it is the experience of "Atonement" with the world and with one's self; it is the end of alienation, the return of man to himself.'[10]

In some instance quoted in the New Testament, Jesus explicitly used inner healing. In the healing of the paralytic we have both an inner and a physical healing (Lk. 5:15-26). Jesus first restored peace to the inner man by forgiving his sins. This healing delivered him from bondage and thus gave him freedom to receive the fullness of life – a complete healing. Then He cured the man of the external symptom, the paralysis, which though real, was symptomatic of the inner bondage.

Today most psychiatrists, psychologists, psychoanalysts and counsellors are aware of the need for inner healing. They spend months and often years probing for traces of

Create Your Own Health Patterns

those deep-rooted emotional scars, realising that there will be no significant growth or change until inner healing takes place.

CONCLUSION

*You were darkness once, but now
you are the light in the Lord;
be like children of light, for
the effects of the light are seen
in complete goodness and right
living and truth.*
EPHESIANS 5: 8-9

As one surveys the world of healing today, one finds quite a variety of concepts and beliefs in relation to healing and a still greater variety of healing techniques. In fact, the belief systems are just about as numerous as the cultural and religious philosophies on which they are based and the techniques by which the healing process is activated are almost as numerous as there are healers. Healing takes place in all cultures, within all belief systems and among all types of people. The fact that healing occurs within a certain belief system or by using a determined healing technique which works, does not justify the conclusion that that is the only valid approach.

I believe that healing can take place in any context, given certain conditions. Fundamental among these conditions are a belief in the possibility of healing together with a desire to be rid of the sickness and a sense of expectancy in relation to the outcome.

I see man as an entity composed of body, mind and spirit and governed by inherent laws which are often referred to as man's nature. Between the different parts of man there is constant interaction and intercommunication. The state of the body can affect the mind and the spirit. A change in the mental state brings about changes in the body and the spirit, and the state of the spirit expresses itself in the mind and in the body. I see good health as the natural consequence of harmonious living where the needs of the differ-

Create Your Own Health Patterns

ent parts of the person are catered for, where the mind, body and spirit work together in an integrated manner for the good of the whole.

On the other hand, I see sickness not as something sent by God, nor even willed by God, but rather as a direct consequence of man's acting contrary to the inherent laws of nature. I understand 'disease' according to the literal meaning of the word – lack of ease, whether it be dis-ease in the mind or dis-ease in the body or dis-ease in a situation. It is an external expression of an internal disharmony or conflict. Some of our conflicts are conscious and are thus more accessible to us, while others are rooted in the subconscious and not so easily available. A particular conflict may be related to self – one's own self image or self acceptance – or may be due to the inability of the person to cope with the environment. It could also be caused by disharmonious social relationships where the flow of love is inhibited or cut off.

In his book, *You Can Heal Yourself*, Dr Masaharu Taniguchi develops a theory that illness comes from wrong thinking linked with inner emotional conflict, and that the only road to permanent good health lies in the re-establishment of complete and total harmony.[1] Man needs to work continually on himself in order to establish inner peace and harmony and he needs to work on his environment in order to make it more conducive to good health.

I understand all healing processes, whether they be psychic healing, faith healing, spiritual healing, or so-called miraculous healing, as natural phenomena, brought about by nature itself and not due to the extraordinary intervention of extrinsic forces and that is why I use the term 'natural healing'. Some see the role of the healer as one of 'mediumship' while others understand it in terms of 'channelling healing energy', or being an 'instrument of Divine Power'. Regardless of the form it may take for people of different belief systems, the healer's function is always one

Create Your Own Health Patterns

of 'mediation'.

In general, we create our own sickness and if we are capable of creating our own sickness then we are capable of re-creating our own health. Once inner peace and harmony are re-established nature has the power to repair itself and good health should ensue.

I see every human being as having the innate ability to heal both self and others. In some this ability is developed to a greater degree. It is an ability which can be enhanced and developed through practice and through the use of certain disciplines.

I consider medical science as a healing approach that is totally inadequate to man's real needs. It is doomed to failure as long as it continues to work within its own limited field. Hence there exists an urgent need for co-operation and understanding between the medical and the non-medical healers.

A healing approach which aims at treating the whole person effecting both an external and internal healing has to be more successful and permanent. Inner healing, which I understand as the re-establishment of peace and harmony within the person, is fundamental for the permanent effective restoration of health.

Acknowledgements

Various people collaborated in the making of this book, and to them I owe a special word of appreciation and gratitude.

David Van Nuys and Eleanor Criswell, my advisors at the Psychology Department of Sonoma State University, who guided me through my studies during a period of two years, and gave me the stimulation and encouragement I needed to embark on the project.

Carol Guion, Associate Editor of the Noetic Sciences Review, Sausalito, California, for her much appreciated editorial assistance.

My friends and colleagues, Patrick Donavan, Patrick Leonard, Ann Coleman, Patrick Peters, Seamus Meagher, Ann Boran and Maria Isabel Cardoso Braga, who read and criticised the original manuscript, and gave extremely valuable suggestions.

Paul Moran, who did the final review and provided the finishing touches to the present edition.

George Boran, who was constantly opening up new horizons, and Hugh Larkin for his sympathetic interest.

Finally Carol Emery and Kethryn Curtis, who provided excellent secretarial assistance, and displayed endless patience in typing and retyping manuscripts.

The author and publisher would like to thank the following for permission to quote material for which they hold the copyright.

The Souvenir Press for material from The Flying Cow by Guy Lyon Playfair; 'Baltimore Spiritual Healers' by Helen Henry, reprinted with permission of the Baltimore Sun Company; Random House for Your Power to Heal by Harold Sherman; Simon and Schuster for The Power of Your Subconscious Mind by Joseph Murphy; Bible text is reproduced from the Good News Bible © American Bible Society, New York, 1966, 1971 and 4th edition 1976, published by The Bible Societies/ Harper Collins, with permission; Scripture text used on page 90 for the Book of Ecclesiasticus (Sirach) is taken from the New American Bible Copyright © 1970 by the Confraternity of Christian Doctrine, Washington, D.C. and is used by permission of the copyright owner. All rights reserved.

NOTES

Chapter I

1. G. L. Playfair, *The Flying Cow*, London, Souvenir Press, 1975.
2. Cf. David St Clair, *Drum and Candle*, London, MacDonald and Co., 1971, p 269.
3. Playfair, *op cit.*, pp 258-259.
4. Helen Hadsell, *The Name It and Claim It Game*, Santa Monica, California, Devors & Co. Publishers, 1971.
5. Hadsell, *ibid*, p 23.

Chapter II

1. Stanley Krippner and Alberto Villoldo, *The Realms of Healing*, Millbrae, California, Celestial Arts, 1976.
2. Quoted by Krippner and Villoldo, p 262.
3. Jerome D. Frank, *Persuasion and Healing*, revised edition, NewYork, Schlocken Books, 1974, p 74.
4. Krippner and Villoldo, *op cit* .
5. Krippner and Villoldo, *op cit.*
6. Harold Sherman, *Your Power to Heal*, Greenwich, Connecticut, Fawcett Publications, Inc., 1972, p 11.
7. *Good News for Foreign Man*, New York, American Bible Society, 1966, 1971 (All further quotes from the New Testament are taken from this edition).
8. Joseph Murphy, *The Power of Your Subconscious Mind*, Englewood Cliffs, New Jersey, Prentice Hall, Inc., 1963, p 56.
9. Joseph Murphy, *ibid* , p 66.
10. Leslie M. Le Cron, *Self Hypnotism,* New York, Prentice Hall 1964.
11. Sherman, *op cit*, p 136.
12. Frank, *op cit.*
13. Frank, *op cit*, p 137.
14. Quoted by Frank, *op cit*, p 136.
15. Frank, *op cit*, p 139.
16. Quoted in A. K. Shapiro, 'The Placebo Effect in the History of Medical Treatment', *American Journal of Psychiatry*, 1959, 116, 298-304.
17. Shapiro, *op cit.*, p 116.
18. Frank, *op cit.*, p 139.
19. F. A. Volgyesi, 'School for patients Hypnosis-Therapy and Psychoprophylaxis', *British Journal of Medical Hypn*osis, 1954, 126:

Create Your Own Health Patterns

1282-89.
20. Frank, *op cit*.
21. S. Wolf and R. H. Pinsky, 'Effects of Placebo Administration and Occurrence of Toxic Reactions', *Journal of American Medical Association*, 1954, 155: 339-41.
22. Clara Thompson, *Psychoanalysis, Evolution and Development*, New York, Hermitage House, 1950.
23. Frank, *op cit*., p 156.
24. *Ibid*.
25. *Ibid*, p 68.
26. *Ibid*.
27. *Ibid*.
28. Ruth Cranston, *The Miracle of Lourdes*, New York, Mc Graw Hill, 1955, p 125.
29. T. C. Everson and W. H. Cole, *Spontaneous Regression of Cancer*, Philadelphia, W. B. Saunders 1966.
30. Frank, *op cit*.
31. *Ibid*.
32. *Encyclopedia Britannica*, Vol. 6, 1973, pp 630-31.
33. Francis MacNutt, *Healing*, Notre Dame, Indiana, Ave Maria Press, 1974, p 41.
34. Viktor Frankl, *Man's Search for Meaning*, Boston, Beacon Press, 1961.
35. MacNutt, *op cit*., p 251.
36. *Ibid*.
37. *Ibid*, p 50.
38. *Ibid*, p 53.

Chapter III

1. David M. Rorvik, 'The Healing Hand of Mr E', *Esquire*, February 1974, p 74.
2. *Ibid*, p 160.
3. Robert N. Miller and Philip B. Reinhart, 'Measuring Psychic Energy', *Psychic*, June 1975.
4. Krippner and Villoldo, *op cit*.
5. Quoted by Krippner and Villoldo, p 99.
6. Quoted by Krippner and Villoldo, p 92.
7. Jack Schwarz, *Human Energy Systems*, New York, E. P. Dutton, 1980.
8. Schwarz, *op cit*.
9. Schwarz, *op cit*.
10. Quoted by Krippner and Villoldo, *op cit*., p 94.
11. *Ibid* p 94.

Create Your Own Health Patterns

12. *Ibid*, p 119.
13. *Ibid*, p 92.
14. Pierre Weil, *A Conscienda Cosmica*, Petropolis, Editora Vozes, 1976, p 68.
15. Schwarz, *op cit*.

Chapter IV

1. *Opiniao*, 10 January 1975, Rio de Janeiro (An adaptation of Ivan Illich's book, *Nemesis Medicale*, published by *Le Nouvel Observateur* and reproduced by *Opiniao*).
2. 'Allocation of Resources to Health', *Journal of Human Resources*, VI, 1971, in *Opiniao*, p 2.
3. *Ibid*.
4. Quoted by *Playboy*, April 1980, Article, 'Medicine and the Mind' by David Black, p 122.
5. *Ibid*.
6. *Ibid*.
7. *Ibid*.
8. John Cassels, Communication to the American Sociological Association, *Opiniao*, 29 August, 1973, p 4.
9. Cf. Black, *op cit*. p 24.
10. J. P. Dupuy and S Karsenty, *Opiniao*, 1974, p 4.
11. Frank, *op cit*.
12. *Ibid*, p 46.
13. Frank, *op cit*., p147.
14. B. Inglis, *The Case for Unorthodox Medicine,*, New York, G. P. Putnam's Sons, 1965, p 53.
15. *Opiniao*, p 5.
16. *San Francisco Chronicle*, 22 July, 1975, p 5.
17. Krippner and Villoldo, *op cit*.
18. *Ibid*.
19. *Ibid*.
20. *Ibid*.
21. *Ibid*.
22. *Ibid*.
23. *Ibid*.
24. *Ibid*.
25. Cf. Black, *op cit*.
26. Krippner and Villoldo, *op cit*.
27. *Ibid*.
28. Quoted by Krippner and Villoldo, *op cit*., p 269.
29. Sherman, *op cit*.
30. MacNutt, *op cit* p 265.

31. Quotation taken from article by Helen Henry, *Baltimore Sun*, 12 December 1965.
32. Quotation from the *New American Bible*, Catholic Book Publishing Co., New York.

Chapter V

1. MacNutt, *op cit.*, p 170.
2. *Ibid*, p 182
3. *Ibid*, p 183.
4. Agnes Stanford, *The Healing Light*, Plainfield, New Jersey, Logos International, 1972.
5. MacNutt, *op cit.*, p 181.
6. Michael Scanlon, *Inner Healing*, New York, Paulist Press, 1974.
7. MacNutt, *op cit.*, p 70.
8. Howard and Martha E. Lewis, *Psychomatics: How Your Emotions Can Damage Your Health*, New York, The Viking Press, 1972, p 7.
9. Howard and Martha Lewis, *op cit.*
10. Erich Fromm, *The Dogma of Christ*, Greenwich, Connecticut, Fawcett Publications, Inc, 1963, pp 187-191.

Conclusion

1. Masaharu Taniguchi, *You Can Heal Yourself*, Tokyo, Seicho-no-ie Foundation, Divine Publication Department, 1961.

BIBLIOGRAPHY

Baltimore Sun, 12 December 1965. Quotation taken from feature article by Helen Henry.
Black, David, 'Medicine and the Mind', *Playboy*, April 1980.

Cassels, John, 'Communication to the American Sociological Association', *Opiniao*, 29 August 1973.
Cranston, Ruth, *The Miracle of Lourdes,* New York, McGraw-Hill 1955.

Dupuy, J. P. and Karsenty, *Opiniao*, 1974.

Everson, T. C. and Cole W. H., *Spontaneous Regression of Cancer*, Philadelphia, W. B. Saunders, 1966.

Frank, Jerome D., *Persuasion and Healing*, revised edition, New York, Schocken Books, 1974.
Frankl, Viktor, *Man's Search for Meaning*, Boston, Beacon Press, 1962.
Fromm, Erich,*The Dogma of Christ*, Greenwich, Connecticut, Fawcett Publications, Inc, 1963.
Fuller, John A Arigo, *Surgeon of the Rusty Knife,* Condensed in Book Section of *Readers Digest*, March 1975.

Good News for Modern Man, Commemorative Edition 1822-1972 New York, American Bible Society.

Hadsell, Helen, *The Name of It and Claim It Game*, Santa Monica, Devors and Co., 1971.

Illich, Ivan, *Nemesis Medicale*, published by *Le Nouvel Observateur* and reproduced by *Opiniao*, 10 January 1975.
Inglis, B, *The Case for Unorthodox Medicine*, New York, G. P. Putnam's Sons, 1965.

Create Your Own Health Patterns

Jerusalem Bible, Copyright 1966 by Dalton Longman and Todd, and Doubleday and Company, Inc.

Kelsey, Morton T, *Healing and Christianity*, New York, Harper and Row, 1973.
Krippner, Stanley and Villoldo, Alberto, *The Realms of Healing*, Millbrae, California, Celestial Arts, 1976.

Le Cron, Leslie M., *Self Hypnotism*, New York, Prentice Hall, Inc., 1964.
Lewis, Howard R. and Martha E, *Psychomatics–How Your Emotions Can Damage Your Health*, New York, The Viking Press, 1972.

MacNutt, Francis, *Healing*, Notre Dame, Ave Maria Press, 1974.
Miller, Robert N. and Reinhart, Philip B., 'Measuring Psychic Energy', *Psychic*, June 1975.
Murphy, Joseph, *The Power of Your Subconscious Mind*, Englewood Cliffs, New Jersey, Prentice-Hall, Inc., 1963.

New American Bible, Catholic Book Publishing Co., New York.
Nouwen, Henry J. M., *The Living Reminder*, New York, The Seabury Press, 1977.

Peale, Norman Vincent, *Power of Positive Thinking*, Englewood Cliffs, New Jersey, Prentice-Hall, Inc.
Playfair, Guy Lyon, *The Flying Cow*, London, Souvenir Press, 1975.

Roberts, Oral, *The Miracle of Seed Faith*, Tulsa, Oral Roberts Publications, 1970.
Rorvik, David M, 'The Healing Hand of Mr E', *Esquire*, February 1974.

San Francisco Chronicle, 22 July 1975.

Scanlon, Michael, *Inner Healing*, New York, Paulist Press, 1974.

Schwarz, Jack, *Human Energy Systems*, New York, E. P. Dutton, 1980.

Shapiro, A. K., 'The Placebo Effect in the History of Medical Treatment', *American Journal of Psychiatry*, 1959, 116: 298-304.

Spragnett, Allen and Kuhlman, Kathryn, *The Woman Who Believes in Miracles*, New York, Thomas E Growall Co., Inc, 1970.

St Clair, David, *Drum and Candle*, London, MacDonald and Co., 1971.

Sherman, Harold, *Your Power to Heal*, Greenwich, Connecticut, Fawcett Publications Inc., 1972.

Stanford, Agnes, *The Healing Light*, Plainfield, New Jersey, Logos International, 1972.

Taniguchi, Masaharu, *You Can Heal Yourself*, Tokyo, Seicho-no-ie Foundation, 1961.

Thompson, Clara, *Psychoanalysis: Evolution and Development*, New York, Hermitage House, 1950.

Volgyesi, F. A., 'School for Patient's Hypnosis-Therapy and Psychoprophylaxis', *British Journal of Medical Hypnosis*, 126: 1282-89, 1954.

Weil, Pierre, *A Conscienda Cosmica*, Petropolis, Editora Vozes, 1976.

Wolf, S and Pinsky, R. H., 'Effects of Placebo Administration and Occurrence of Toxic Reactions', *Journal of American Medical Association* , 155: 339-341, 1954.

More Interesting Titles

Body-Mind Meditation
A Gateway to Spirituality

Louis Hughes, OP

You can take this book as your guide for a fascinating journey that need not take you beyond your own hall door. For it is an inward journey, and it will take you no further than God who, for those who want him as a friend, lives within. On the way to God-awareness, you will be invited to experience deep relaxation of body and mind.

Body-Mind Meditation can help you become a more integrated balanced person. It is an especially helpful approach to meditation if the pace of life is too fast for you, or if you find yourself frequently tense or exhausted.

SPIRITUALITY AND HOLISTIC LIVING

Sr. Theresa Feist

You are in search of wholeness. You have a body, mind and spiritual life. Your spirit cannot soar if your feet are heavy. Your mind is confused when your blood is stagnant. You need to care properly for your temple.

An Easy Guide to Meditation

Roy Eugene Davis

Meditation is the natural process to use to release tension, reduce stress, increase awareness, concentrate more effectively and be open to life. In this book you will learn how to meditate correctly for inner growth and spiritual awareness. Specific guidelines are provided to assist the beginner as well as the more advanced meditator. Here are proven techniques used by accomplished meditators for years: *prayer, mantra, sound–light contemplation, ways to expand consciousness and to experience transcendence.*

Benefits of correct meditation practice include: deep relaxation, stress reduction, inner calm, improved powers of intelligence, and strengthening of the immune system. People in all walks of life can find here the keys to living life as it was meant to be lived.

An Easy Guide to Meditation was written by one who knows how to meditate and who, for decades, has been teaching the process to thousands of people all over the world. Roy Eugene Davis has written many other books including *Our Awakening World, Secrets of Inner Power, With God We Can* and *God Has Given Us Every Good Thing.*

Over 100,000 copies sold.

THE GIFT OF MIRACLES
Experiencing God's Extraordinary Power in Your Life
Robert DeGrandis, SSJ
with Linda Schubert

- A woman is healed of epilepsy after fourteen years of seizures
- A severely retarded ten-month-old baby boy dies of infant flu, and returns to life perfectly normal!

This wonderful gift of miracles is being poured out today – as in the time of the early Christians and the lives of the saints – if we will only open our eyes to see, insists Fr Robert DeGrandis. In *The Gift of Miracles*, he recounts these and dozens of other miracles from his many years of ministry.

Here are the testimonies of modern-day miracles worked through the sacraments, the intercession of Mary, and the expectant prayer in everyday life. Fr DeGrandis has also included practical tips and model prayers to use when you are interceding for healing and miracles.

The Gift of Miracles will not only inspire you and those you love, but encourage you to expect the miraculous in your life

PETER CALVAY HERMIT

Rayner Torkington

This is a fast moving and fascinating story of a young priest in search of holiness and of the hermit who helps him. The principles of Christian Spirituality are pinpointed with a ruthless accuracy that challenges the integrity of the reader, and dares him to abandon himself to the only One who can radically make him new. The author not only shows how prayer is the principal means of doing this, but he details a 'Blue Print' for prayer for the beginner, and outlines and explains the most ancient Christian prayer tradition, while maintaining the same compelling style throughout.

Over 34,000 copies of this bestseller have been sold.

PETER CALVAY PROPHET

Rayner Torkington

This book is first and foremost a brilliant exposition of the inner meaning of prayer and of the profound truths that underlie the spiritual life. Here at last is a voice that speaks with authority and consumate clarity amidst so much contemporary confusion, of the only One who makes all things new and of how to receive Him.

THE WAY OF A HEALER

Peter Gill

Introduction by Lilla Bek

THE WAY OF A HEALER deals with different aspects of healing, and the way that spiritual healing works in the lives of people. Healing means health, and health is wholeness. That word wholeness implies a number of separate parts coming together to make a complete whole. We are accustomed to the concept of body, mind and soul, and unless these different aspects of ourselves function together in harmony we have disharmony or dis-ease. If that condition of dis-ease is allowed to continue unchecked, ultimately we have disease or illness. Spiritual healing works at the physical, mental, emotional and spiritual levels of a person.

Today we stand upon the brink of the darkest age that could yet befall mankind, or, with a change of consciousness, upon the edge of a new and wonderful dawn to herald in a golden age. What that age will be depends upon what we make of it now. The immediate need is for a concept which will integrate us with the life of the solar system and, through the solar consciousness, link us with the life of the universe and the word of God. Our thinking must become much more expansive to embrace, not only humankind as we know it, but also the angel, elemental and nature kingdoms, and other realms not normally perceived by our physical sense.